Easy Potpourri

David A. Webb

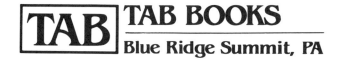
TAB BOOKS
Blue Ridge Summit, PA

Dedicated to
Charles, Robert, Merry,
and my mother, Marion.

FIRST EDITION
FIRST PRINTING

© 1992 by **TAB Books**.
TAB Books is a division of McGraw-Hill, Inc.

Library of Congress Cataloging-in-Publication Data

Webb, David A.
Easy potpourri / by David A. Webb.
p. cm.
Includes index.
ISBN 0-8306-2128-8   ISBN 0-8306-2127-X (pbk.)
1. Perfumes. 2. Potpourris (Scented floral mixtures) I. Title.
TP983.W343 1991   91-12051
745.92—dc20   CIP

Acquisitions Editor: Kimberly Tabor
Book Editor: April D. Nolan
Production: Katherine G. Brown
Book Design: Jaclyn J. Boone
Page Makeup: Toya B. Warner
Cover Photo: Susan Riley, Harrisonburg, VA
Cover: Holberg Design, York, PA

Contents

_____PART THREE_____

Heated Fragrances

——————————————————PART FOUR——————————————————
Colognes & Soaps

————————————————PART FIVE————————————————
Crafts for Today's Lifestyle

Acknowledgments

I WOULD LIKE TO THANK the following people and organizations for the help they provided:

Marion Michaels, Black River Falls, Wisconsin.
Merry Michaels, Black River Falls, Wisconsin.
Charles Webb, Chippewa Falls, Wisconsin.
Mary Borofka-Webb, Chippewa Falls, Wisconsin.
Dr. Robert I. Webb, Charlottesville, Virginia.
Mary Beth Webb, Charlottesville, Virginia.
Elizabeth Brümmer, German Information Center, New York.
Embassy of the People's Republic of China, Washington, D.C.
Star Przybilla, Hixton, Wisconsin.
Debra Dawn Rasmussen, Minneapolis, Minnesota.
Embassy of India, Washington, D.C.
Myrtle Doud, Black River Falls, Wisconsin.
Doris Erhardt, Fort Wayne, Indiana.
Elizabeth Spangler, Black River Falls, Wisconsin.
Alvalina Nandory, Black River Falls, Wisconsin.
Embassy of Turkey, Washington, D.C.
Charles Webb Sr., Brooklyn, New York.
Thomas Webb, Brooklyn, New York.

Introduction

THIS BOOK IS FOR PEOPLE whose latent creative abilities are bubbling to the surface, who love nature in all its aromatic glory, who despise the superabundance of artificial chemicals in many commercial products, and who desire luxurious items to use and to give.

Easy Potpourri is an easy-to-understand reference guide. All "recipes" use the familiar English standards. Although the formulas in this book are called "recipes," this analogy might be somewhat misleading. Making soap, candles, colognes, etc., is not the same as cooking or baking. In ordinary culinary endeavors, you can place a pot on the stove and go about other chores while it cooks. You can place a cake in the oven, set the temperature control, and return later. Don't try that with soap! Even baking a cake depends upon the individual oven. In some ovens a cake will come out raw in the middle; in others, it might be overcooked; in some, it's charred around the edges—all baked for the same exact period of time!

The formulas in this book require your full and undivided attention. You *cannot* manufacture soap and just go about your routine chores at the same time!

All recipes in this book can be made in about one hour, but there are many variables to consider. For example, it takes several days to soak wood ashes to make lye. Also, water differs in its mineral content and, consequently, in how rapidly it boils. Many variations affect cooking pressures and times—altitude, your own stove's idiosyncracies and speed of cooking, the hardness of the final product you desire and the size batch you're making, to name a few.

In researching this book, everyone I interviewed stressed that time is not an accurate tool of measurement for making soap, candles, and colognes. The hour figures mentioned here are meant to be estimates, not standards of measurement. *Saponification*, the conversion of fat into soap, is a chemical reaction. It does not occur according to a precise time-table, and certainly not in the home kitchen. The simple fats do not combine with alkali to form soap, but are first decomposed to form fatty acids and glycerols. When you are dealing with nature, remember that no two of anything are exactly alike; we all know that each snowflake is unique. But this doesn't mean you can't work with natural ingredients. Just as a chef often tastes a special soup, so will you check your mixture for consistency and "feel."

Whenever you decide to work any of the formulas in this book, it is necessary to set aside ample time to do the job. Working in blocks of time often produces the best results. Select a couple of hours of the day (or night) when you will not be disturbed. Take your phone off the hook and turn off the TV so there are no distractions.

Soap making was a necessary craft for the pioneers, and they didn't have paint-by-number kits for creating their natural products. Likewise, most of us interested in these basic activities today don't want to be led around by the hand. Instead, we want our creativity, our unique input to show. Soap making is partly a science and partly an art. Your skills will vastly improve with practice.

Easy Potpourri provides a wealth of information for the person interested in these exciting home crafts. Chapter 1 outlines the many reasons why people choose to make their own potpourris, homemade soaps, etc. Reasons vary from simple hobby interests to ethical principles. Chapter 2 discusses the tools and equipment needed to make the various items in this book. These include such instruments as mortar and pestle (for grinding fresh herbs) to tools for making colognes to the safety eye goggles absolutely essential for making soap.

Chapter 3 explores English potpourri. It includes the history of some flowers, such as the Red Rose of Lancaster. It has a unique quality in that its petals retain their heady perfume even when dried, which makes it ideal for potpourris and sachets. If you are an Anglophile, you will enjoy the recipe for Rue and Rosemary potpourri. These scents were extremely popular during the reign of Queen Victoria.

Chapter 4 introduces you to European potpourris. Potpourri was invented in France, and many French potpourris have as ingredients roses that were grown in Empress Josephine's famous rose garden at Malmaison. Chapter 5 travels to the Orient and lets you experience the exotic fragrances native to India, Sri Lanka, China, and Japan.

Chapter 6 shows you how to make dream pillows, a custom of several Native American tribes. These pillows were small pouches filled with native herbs and botanicals that, when laid close to the sleeper's face at night, were said to help the sleeper achieve vivid dreams. Other exciting Americana projects are included, as well as directions for making potpourris for your pets.

Chapter 7 is filled with Christmas projects that your whole family will enjoy making, and chapter 8 concerns the hot potpourris that have become quite popular recently. Chapter 9 shows you how to make scented candles using beeswax, candlewick, or your favorite candlemolds to create scented candles for home or for gifts.

Chapter 10 examines how incense is made. Incense burning is regaining in popularity. The information on making "Ghee" and its uses should be of special interest to those interested in the philosophies of India.

Chapter 11 presents the fascinating art of cologne making as a home craft. Be sure to check out the brief history of *eau de cologne*, with its origin in the city of Cologne (Köln), Germany, and how the original "toilet waters" have evolved into colognes we know today. Colognes should always be packaged attractively whether used for gifts or sales.

Chapter 12 is filled with Oriental colognes. Of special interest are the Tibetan recipes. Because musk is used in the manufacture of perfume, I suggest using synthetic musk oil if you object to the use of animal extracts. Colognes from Tibet rely heavily on this scent.

Chapter 13 presents the pioneer art of soap making. I have provided many soap formulas, all tried and tested. I've used the commercial brand, Lewis Lye for my soaps, but other brands should be equally suitable for the task. Remember: Making homemade soaps requires a great deal of patience, as well as your full and undivided attention, but it is certainly a rewarding craft once mastered.

Chapter 14 examines unusual soaps. Of special interest are the fruit-shaped soaps of Turkey. These are no longer made because modern culture has reduced the interest in these old crafts, but such soaps are still found in museums. Chapter 15 is for people who have limits to their time and patience. There are many handy shortcuts for busy people who still want to create something of their own. Check out the quick potpourris.

Chapter 16 discusses a popular pastime—making money! Even if a great deal of love and skill go into making your homecrafts, unless you know how to market them, they might not make money for you. Everyone, of course, is not interested in selling their scented creations, but things of value are always in demand.

Easy Potpourri gives you an opportunity to try your skills at creating fragrances from places far and near—to imagine, with the aid of the scents of yesteryear, what life might have been like in the Royal Gardens of France, or in the Royal Gardens at the palace of Yuanyuanming, China, before it was burned down by the British and French Forces.

This is one "recipe" book you'll treasure. Even people concerned about animal suffering can enjoy fragrances that resemble old European favorites because no animal extractions are used in any of the formulas. With this book you'll be able to enjoy the scents of spring and summer even in the gray chill of winter. Your own aromatic potpourris, sensual colognes, and wonderful soaps will tantalize your senses all year long, pleasing relatives and friends, and possibly even customers.

Part 1

The
Basics

Chapter 1

Why Make Your Own?

EVERY INDIVIDUAL needs to express the part of him or herself that is unique to that individual. According to Maslow's Hierarchy of Needs, the need for self-actualization exists on a higher level, and creativity is part of the self-actualization process. You might have noticed that the happiest people are often the most creative. You might not have realized before that a link exists between happiness and creative expression, but it does.

Satisfying the human need to be creative is one of the reasons behind the popularity of do-it-yourself crafts and projects. Most of us have too long neglected our creative natures. Imagine a preschooler who makes fantastic works of art and then starts school, only to have her imagination and creativity dulled after repeated insistence on "coloring within the lines." As adults, we often face a life of punching clocks and doing repetitive tasks. We need to be more attuned to our inner selves for our creativity to again blossom, and do-it-yourself projects—especially of the pleasing nature of potpourris, colognes, incense, special soaps, and candles—can be just what we need to inspire our imagination.

Some people have such well-developed imaginations that they can create things entirely from scratch. Most people, however, do best when they have some framework or guidelines. Following a tried and true recipe or blueprint is most practical. When properly executed, these plans ensure success. Every success grows, building skills in that area. It is often said that people learn from their mistakes, but that is only half true. People also learn from their successes. In fact, if they spend too much time studying their mistakes, they will only develop higher skills for blunder.

Whenever you create something, the resulting product is endowed with a special value, most often lost in factory production. You will discover that the finest crafts are those that have been crafted with love, using individual ingenuity.

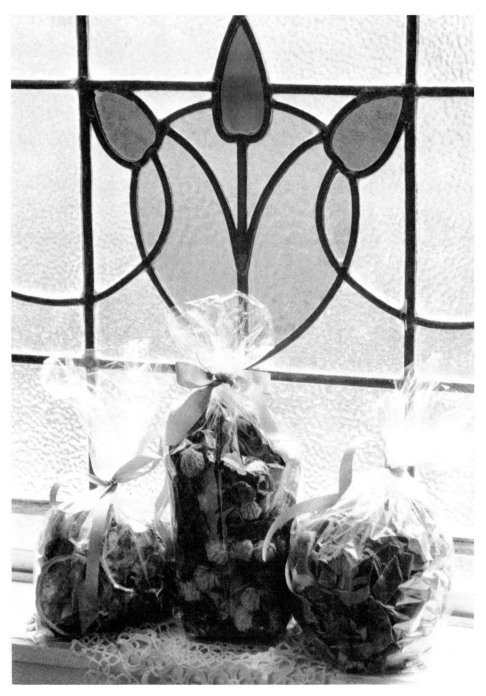

Creativity can blossom through do-it-yourself projects such as making homemade potpourri.

ONE-OF-A-KIND CREATIONS

Rediscovering and using your own creativity isn't the only reason for making your own fragrant products. One of the most important reasons is that you'll be making products that are original and exclusive—products that aren't available to just anyone.

You might be able to buy a bar of soap at a cost comparable to (or even less than) the expense you incur in making your own. But when you consider quality, dollar for dollar, making your own is an excellent investment. If you have ever priced the top-notch perfumes on the market, you know precisely what I mean. When you do it yourself, you can luxuriate in "Mercedes-Benz" or "Rolls-Royce" fragrances as you soak in your one-of-a-kind bubble bath. Or you can splash on a cologne of essences combined to satisfy your personal pleasure and aesthetics, the like of which cannot be found drawing dust on some drugstore counter. Your creations are yours exclusively and are, therefore, unique.

When you consider what you would have to pay someone to create a product especially for you or your friends, you can feel as rich as royalty because you'll know you have saved a bundle.

HARD-TO-FIND PRODUCTS

A good argument for creating your own is that often what you want cannot be found in the marketplace. Many stores stock only a limited number of potpourris, colognes, and soaps. These products are usually available because they are part of a stock line offered by the store's suppliers or because they are good sellers in the area. Either way the results can be frustrating to you as a consumer.

Because most stores carry only certain brands, you might have to travel some distance to find the store that offers you what you want. Stores that stock only fast-selling items also limit your choices to items currently popular in your area, and you might not share in transient fads.

Specialty Mail Order

If you can't find the items you seek locally, you might want to consider another route. Specialty mail-order companies offer many unusual and hard-to-find products, and they can be an excellent source for that rare potpourri, cologne, or soap you really want. Mail-order companies usually have a larger inventory than local stores, and they usually don't limit their selection to name brands.

Mail-order companies offer other advantages. For example, the convenience of shopping at home can save you the gas you would waste running around town to find what you want. However, mail order has two big disadvantages: time and money. Anything that you order by mail will take much more time to get to you than something you pick up at a store. In addition, there's nothing worse than waiting weeks for your order to arrive, only to find out it's out of stock and on back order, indicating another long wait.

Money can be another obstacle. Mail-order goods are often more expensive than similar goods purchased locally. Sometimes they are substantially higher, especially when ordered from specialty catalogs. To get what you want, you often have to pay more than you'd like.

Making Your Own

Obviously, if you want one-of-a-kind creations, the best alternative is to make your own. When you make you own, you aren't at the mercy of what's popular, and you aren't stuck with an item because it's the only one the store carries. You don't have to wait for weeks or months for your package to arrive in the mail. When you make your own, you spare yourself many frustrations.

Perhaps one of the most important reasons to do it yourself is the money you'll save. You can make quality products yourself without paying exorbitant prices and wasting time looking for something unique.

QUALITY CONTROL

There was a time when products were made with ingredients that you could identify and read. That time has long past. Look at any label and you're likely to read a long list of chemicals. Many of these chemicals have names you can't pronounce. Other ingredients might leave you wondering what their purpose is or where they come from. You wonder, is this safe? Or will it appear as a possible carcinogen on some governmental list a month from now? It's scary!

When you make your own potpourris, colognes, and soaps, you know what is going into your recipes because you are in charge of production from start to finish. There are no unpleasant surprises; you can familiarize yourself with the ingredients and omit anything you don't trust. You can leave out certain harsh ingredients and poisonous additives. You can blend in oils of real flowers, trees, or herbs—even rose petals in some products. You can decide to use lemons or lemon juice when a commercial product might choose a cheaper, less natural acid.

You can also select your personal favorites for ingredients—lilies of the valley or roses, for example—or even the fragrances most loved by your friends, your mother, and others.

Making a Personal Ecological Statement

With the widening hole in the ozone and the serious pollution that plagues our world, more people are becoming aware of the delicate balance of nature. People are beginning to accept individual responsibility for their environment and to take personal action. Individual acts might not seem important, but when millions of individuals start committing themselves to a better environment, the results can be dramatic.

Whether your concern is land dumps, hazardous chemicals, nuclear waste, or animal rights, there are steps that you as an individual can take.

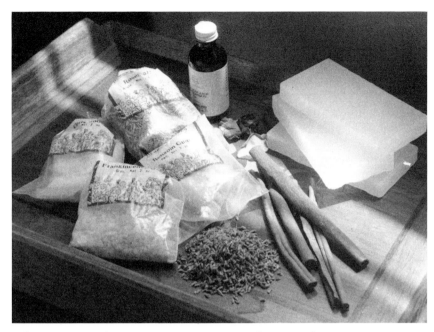

When you make your own, you can choose what goes into your product—and what stays out.

One step you can take for animal rights is to use synthetic musk oil.

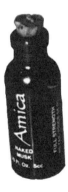

One step involves the choices you make. You can make a choice to change the world. Questionable chemicals are often used in commercial products because they are cheap for manufacturers to use. The same thing can be said of animal fats and other by-products of slaughterhouses.

When you make your own, you can substitute vegetable fats for animal fats, and avoid using harsh chemicals. By making your own, you keep out garbage and questionable fillers from your finished product. There is great satisfaction in knowing what went into a product. You'll breathe easier knowing that family and friends can use your product safely.

FAMILY PROJECTS

In today's busy work world, many parents are concerned about not spending enough time with their children and spouses. As a result, many of us try to make the most of the time our families spend together. There is a certain merit to the concept of "quality time" (although it has been the unfortunate butt of many jokes). Family projects offer a good way for people to spend quality time with their children and spouses. Creative crafts help create a sense of unity and closeness among family members, the same "spirit" people get from being part of a team. Relationships between friends, also, can be strengthened by working together.

Children are not the mindless idiots that so many adults believe them to be. Contrary to many myths, unfortunately perpetuated by television sitcoms, children can and will be constructive, and they actually enjoy doing creative activities. Remember, though, that kids have a shorter attention span than adults. Schedule activities to hold your children's interest. Younger children usually won't want to work continuously on a project for as long as older children will. If you see them start to lose interest, release them to do other things. Do it *before* they start getting bored and goofing off, and thank them enthusiastically for what they did.

Be sure to make the family project something special. Be excited and enthusiastic so family members will look forward to it. Don't make it a grueling ordeal or nobody, including yourself, will want to partake of it for long.

Grownups often forget that neither children nor adults are born with knowledge. All people must grow by learning. If a child makes an error, don't heavily scold or criticize him. Point out something he did right, then, show him the correct way to do the job. You might say, for example, "You picked the perfect color," or "You almost got it," or "That was a great first try." In the end, if necessary, let your child produce an imperfect product, lopsided, top-heavy, or whatever. Grandma or Grandpa will still love it, and so will you.

If children look upset or discouraged, tell them they gave it a good try. Words of encouragement will bolster their self-confidence. Words of criticism will make them feel inadequate and resentful. Don't forget to praise them lavishly and specifically when they really do a good job.

Selecting Family Projects

When you select a family project, keep the ages of your children in mind. Never try complicated or risky projects with young children. Soap making is not for preschoolers, but young children can help in making potpourris. Making colognes may have a special appeal to your teens: Teenage boys often experiment with aftershaves and colognes, and teenage girls like to sample various perfumes and colognes.

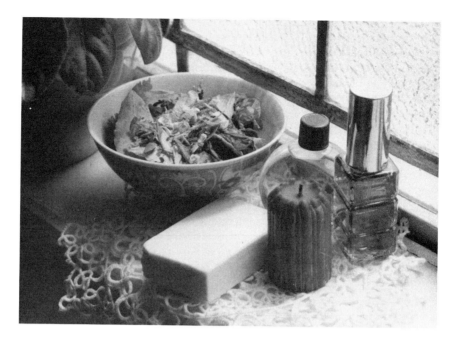

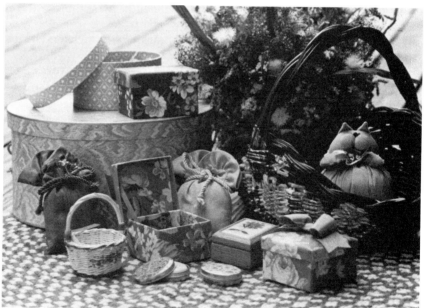

Fragrant homemade products make special gifts with a personal touch.

Don't forget grandparents and other adults when planning family projects. Extended family involvement helps to develop closer family ties and to counter peer pressure, which is especially important as your children mature. Statistics show that children with strong family bonds are less likely to be involved with drugs, alcohol, or experimental sex.

Although television has its merits, too often children as well as other family members, become "couch potatoes." By stimulating interest in worthwhile activities you can stretch the imagination of your youngsters. Creative people are never bored. You have no doubt seen many children who are so accustomed to being entertained all the time that they expect life to be a constant three-ring circus. Those children easily become bored and obnoxious as they seek the attention and respect they crave. The best way to have fun is to create it. The younger your children are when they learn that lesson, the better.

Family bonds are strengthened when you spend time doing things together. Making potpourris can be great fun for young children, making colognes will hold teens' interest, and soap making will fascinate older family members.

GIFT GIVING

There are few pleasures as rewarding as bestowing a gift to a loved one or friend. An even greater pleasure is when the gift is something you created! Homemade potpourris, colognes, and soaps are a special way to show your love. They offer a personal touch that will be appreciated by the recipient.

Store-bought gifts will pale in comparison to your homemade potpourris. Friends and relatives will delight in these treasures from your garden. As time goes by, your gifts will remain as fond memories of you.

Making Gifts Special

The gift that is really special is the one that comes from the heart. It is the gift into which you have put careful thought and effort. Remember the gifts that you cherish? The scarf mother knitted for you, the afghan your aunt Doris made for you. The most important ingredient of any gift is love.

Put extra effort into your homemade products so that they are something you're actually proud of. Don't give away items that you've botched up. Quality is always appreciated; junk isn't.

Wrap gifts with special papers and ribbons. The way you wrap a gift often reveals what you think of the gift and how you feel towards the recipient. The Japanese go to great lengths in wrapping gifts. In Japan, gift-wrapping is an art form, and the wrap often becomes as important as the gift itself. While you might not want to go to the elaborate steps the Japanese do, you should still take time to wrap items nicely. After all the time you've invested in your product, you won't want to skimp on the wrappings.

Use some forethought when selecting gifts. If Grandpa never uses cologne, try giving him soap instead. It will spare hurt feelings later if you actually give him something that he will enjoy. It's also a good idea to acquaint yourself to what scents the person likes. Never assume that because you like a scent, everyone else does, too. Spicy colognes are popular for men, but not all men like them. Choose your gifts for the individual, not for some social stereotype.

One complaint many women voice is that men always assume that they like roses. Many women do, as do many men. However, people are different. The best gift shows a sensitivity to the recipient's desires.

SUPPLEMENTING YOUR INCOME

Who wouldn't enjoy have a few extra dollars? Making money is fun. And when you earn money by doing something that you truly enjoy, then you are living in the best of all possible worlds.

The two factors that will make the difference for you are time and commitment. You must take time to engage in any business, even a part-time one. You must also make a commitment to the quality of your product, and to the satisfaction of your customers.

A Secret To Success

Any business can be successful as long as it attracts satisfied customers. Catering to your customers wants and desires should be your top priority. The most successful businesses are those which serve the needs of your clients. See chapter 16 for more ideas on marketing.

Chapter 2

How to Begin

MANY OF THE TOOLS you need to prepare potpourris, colognes, and soaps are commonplace items you should have around the house, while others are unique to the craft and have to be purchased specially. Regardless, you should always set aside specific tools for their specific tasks. Tools that are used for multiple purposes often get lost or dirty, and they're not always accessible when you need them.

In addition, keeping tools for one intended purpose can help you avoid dangerous mistakes. For example, you should never mix up kettles used for soap making with pots used for cooking meals! While some items—a kitchen scale, for example—lend themselves easily to a multiplicity of uses, most tools do not and should be restricted in their applied use.

TOOLS TO MAKE POTPOURRI

Bowl and Spoon. A large stainless steel bowl and a large wooden spoon are very useful in making potpourri. You can use a glass or ceramic bowl as a substitute, but avoid using plastic bowls; they have a tendency to absorb odors. Likewise, you can use steel spoons instead of wood, but be careful not to crush your ingredients as you stir. You could spoil their aesthetic appeal, as in crushing rosebuds.

It is very important to wash the spoon and bowl thoroughly after each use so they don't transfer the scents of one batch of potpourri to another. If you use bleach or a strongly scented detergent, be certain to rinse them off well to eliminate any of their residual odor. Potpourri is very sensitive; it often picks up odors adding to its bouquet, so be sure detergent or bleach aren't among the odors your potpourri picks up.

Your bowl and spoon should always be large, even if you are preparing a small batch of potpourri. The better the ingredients are mixed, the higher the quality of potpourri will be, and it's much easier to mix ingredients in a large bowl.

Kitchen Scale. You might want to invest in a kitchen scale if you don't already have one. If you make large batches or are following old recipes, weight measures can be crucial to your success. If you are producing potpourris for commercial sale, a scale is essential because most of the ingredients you will buy are sold in weight measures—ounces, pounds, etc. You'll also be able to know exactly what your real production costs are if you keep track of exactly how much you are using.

Naturally, for home or gift purposes, exact weights are not as important. You might rely on "smidgeons" or "dashes," provided that you maintain the proper proportions of your ingredients.

Eyedropper. You should have an eyedropper to measure essential oils and other liquid ingredients. Whenever you add essential oils to a potpourri, you only need a drop or two. Any more and the potpourri will lose its bouquet. **Note:** Keep this dropper separate from any other so that it is never accidentally used in your eyes!

Mortar and Pestle. Although they are not essential to potpourri-making, many people enjoy using a mortar and pestle. A *mortar* is a small marble or ceramic bowl, polished except for the inside bottom. A *pestle* is a marble or a wooden stick, polished except for the rounded end, which is left rough to grind herbs and spices in the mortar. These tools are handy for those who like to employ fresh herbs or spices in their potpourri. If you are accustomed to using powdered spices, a mortar and pestle aren't necessary, but they can be a good investment if you need to grind herbs.

Containers. Don't forget the containers! After you've completed your potpourris, you will need containers to put them in. You can make containers from numerous materials, or you can buy many decorative and unique containers in craft or specialty stores.

The most important consideration in your selection of containers is that they should be functional, yet attractive. Glass or ceramic containers should have some area where the aroma of the potpourri can penetrate. You can use covered containers with removable or vented lids. See-through containers can be attractive; they allow the aesthetic qualities of the potpourri to be appreciated along with the fragrant qualities.

TOOLS AND MATERIALS FOR COLOGNE MAKING

As with making potpourri, you'll need a large stainless steel or glass bowl to make cologne. You'll also need an eyedropper and a funnel. These items are things you probably have around the house.

Still. You can purchase perfume-making kits that include stills for making alcohol. However, I recommend that you save money by purchasing distilled water and alcohol over the counter.

Distilled Water. *Distilled water* is water that has been vaporized as steam and then cooled to condense as water again. It is important to use

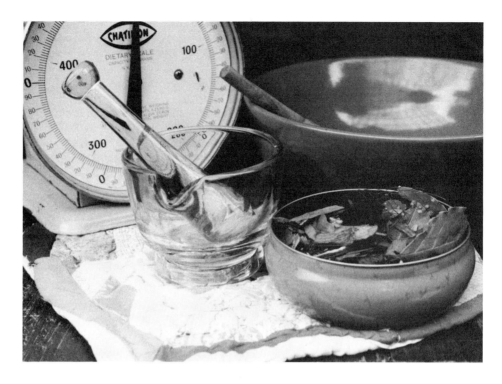

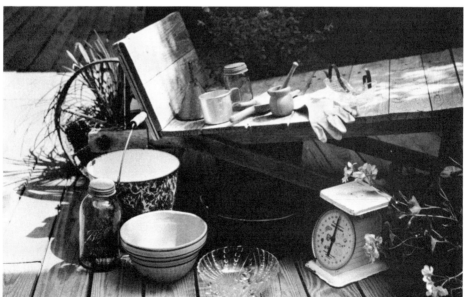

Some common tools will help in preparing potpourri.

only distilled water when making colognes because regular tap water might contain impurities or chlorine which will adversely affect the quality of your colognes.

Alcohol. The type of alcohol you use will also affect the quality of your colognes. The higher the concentration of alcohol, known as *proof*, the more effective it will be in your cologne. Colognes that are used in the ordinary manner—that is, externally—may be made with unscented rubbing alcohol, a very economical and quite efficient alternative to making your own alcohol in a still.

Colognes used in cooking, or in making cakes, frostings, or pastries *must* be made with beverage-grade alcohols only. Never mix the two uses! Always keep edible colognes separate from regular colognes.

If available, alcohol from grapes is preferred above all others. Grapes contain *oeanthic ether*, which makes for the best perfumes. This is where owning your own still can come in handy: you can make your own alcohol from grapes.

Containers. When selecting containers for your colognes choose attractive bottles with a tight seal, so the cologne doesn't evaporate. Small bottles are more practical than large ones. You might want to order bottles specifically made for colognes from a specialty store. You can use an old gallon milk jug for storing colognes, but never use them as a final container. It really isn't civil to present someone with a gallon of cologne! The recipient might take offense.

Remember also that colognes are best stored away from heat and out of direct sunlight. Darkened containers are preferrable to clear ones. Light will degrade a cologne over a period of time, as will excessive heat. Store all colognes in a cool, dry location.

TOOLS FOR SOAP MAKING

The common tools you need to make soap include a measuring cup, a kitchen scale, and a large wooden spoon. Never use the tools you make soap with for other purposes, with the possible exception of the kitchen scale.

Large Kettle. Don't attempt to make soap in a small pan, not even for making small batches. Always use a kettle sufficiently large enough to hold the hot mixture without it boiling over. Use only a large *wooden* spoon for stirring. This is very important, because soap gets very hot. The heat from the hot soap will transfer to the spoon. If a metal spoon is used, the handle will quickly become too hot to touch.

Safety Eye Goggles. One tool that is absolutely essential is a pair of safety goggles. Never attempt to make soap without eye protection. Dangerous gases are released in the saponification (soap making) process that can cause injury and even blindness. It is imperative that everyone in the room where the soap is being made wears safety goggles.

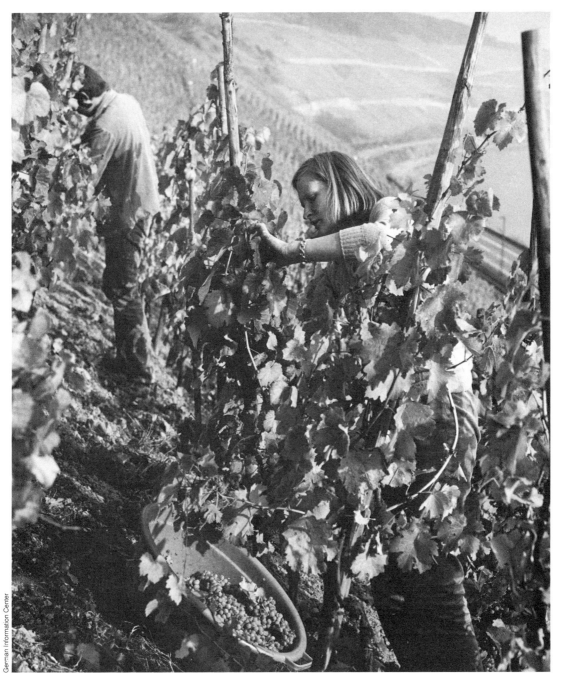

German Information Center

Grapes make the best alcohol for use in cologne.

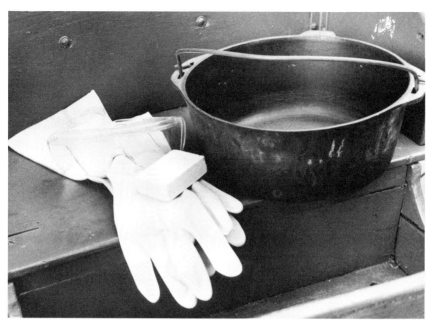

Soap making requires both special tools and special attention.

TOOL CARE

Taking proper care of your tools is an art in itself. First, and foremost, tools should always be used for the purpose to which they were intended. Tools used for other purposes often end up broken.

To make tools work efficiently, to make them last, to prevent accidents, keep tools clean. Keeping tools requires keeping them clean. Cleanliness is vital to the success of your potpourris, colognes, and soaps. Dirty utensils can harbor bacteria or other harmful pathogens that will adversely affect your scented products. Bacteria can cause potpourris to rot or mold, shortening their timespan and sometimes resulting in the stench of rotting flowers and herbs.

Always work with clean tools and clean hands. You can wear rubber gloves, but wash them after each use with soap and water to keep bacteria out of your scented products.

Store Tools Safely

Always keep tools in a secure place to make it easy to find them when you need them. Keeping tools in order can be very time-saving when you are looking for them. Tools kept in a chaotic fashion will be difficult to locate when you need them.

Store tools in a safe, dry location that is secure from children and pets. Cats and dogs are especially curious animals. They take interest in all

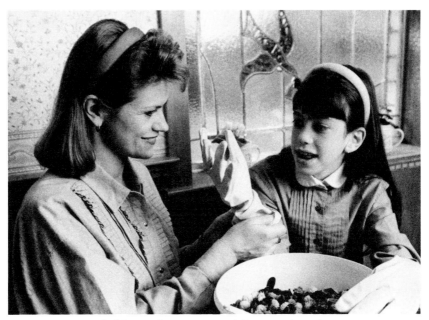

Teach young children the responsible use of tools.

sorts of things. If your pet decides to walk off with a tool, you might not find that tool for days.

Children also play with tools. They break tools unintentionally, and sometimes hurt themselves or others. Keep tools out of the reach of small hands. Teach children the responsible use of tools, and don't horse around with them yourself. Setting a good example is the best teaching method.

SEARCHING OUT SUBSTITUTES

Freshly dried flowers are not always available. Sometimes the herbs you desire cannot be found. For these and other reasons, you might find substitutes useful. It might not be practical to substitute for a main ingredient in a potpourri, but it's not impossible. A rose-scented potpourri can be made without any roses! Certain herbs produce a reasonable facsimile in many instances. For example, you can use lemongrass in place of lemon oil or lemon peel to provide the fragrance of lemon your recipe calls for. A number of geraniums come in rose, lemon, fruit, and spice scents and have been used since time immemorial in quality potpourris.

Creating Illusion

One of the tricks of substitution is the knowledge that you are creating an illusion. Substitute flowers or herbs can provide color and bulk to a potpourri. The illusion isn't so difficult to master when you realize that all dried flowers and herbs lose some of their resemblance to the fresh. A close-up examination might reveal an imposter, but people rarely examine things that closely. In fact, most people generally accept things as true to their description (within reason).

However, keep in mind that scented products made with substitutes for commercial purposes should be labeled with a disclaimer. The disclaimer should state "imitation" rose potpourri, or "artificial" lemon-scented soap. Often ingredients are listed on a product's label in order of ingredient proportion. This information is provided on labels for consumer protection. Just as when we buy apple juice we expect the real thing, if something is labeled "imitation" or "artificial," we know what we are buying.

Some flowers make excellent substitutes for others. For example, dried rose-form begonias resemble rosebuds. And dried peony petals can be used to create the illusion of rose petals. Fragrances have to be added from elsewhere, either from herbs or essential oils. Avoid flowers that are highly scented unless you can easily mask their scent.

Herbs might be more difficult to substitute. If the essential oil of your favorite herb is not available, you can select a substitute that doesn't have much odor of its own. A drop or two of the essential oil of the original, and nobody will be the wiser.

It is important to remember that potpourris are blends. You needn't mask totally the scent of the substitute. If you do, you might overpower the potpourri and destroy the bouquet of blended fragrances that is the hallmark of a good potpourri.

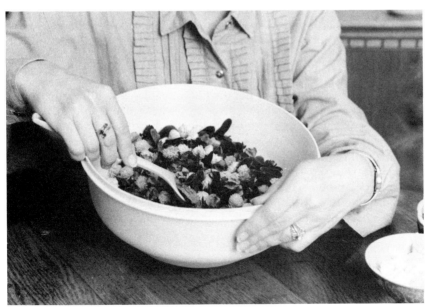

Stir carefully so you don't crush ingredients.

Color is another factor to consider when selecting suitable substitutes. Most rose potpourris are expected to have red or pink in them. Although there are yellow roses, white roses, and roses in many different hues, the public will react with skepticism if a potpourri doesn't look like what they expect. Part of the success of illusion is the attempt to meet people's expectations.

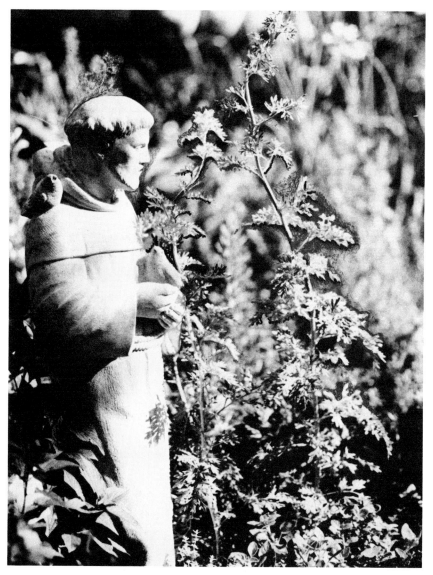

You can substitute flowers or herbs for those the recipe calls for in order to add bulk to a potpourri.

Aesthetic Considerations

I can't emphasize aesthetic considerations strongly enough, especially if you're dealing in commercial sales. Unattractive products will fetch less money in the marketplace—it's that simple. Although commercial food-grade dyes are available at most supermarkets, you might prefer to avoid them because if you label potpourris "artificially-colored," it might hurt sales among the growing number of ecologically concerned people. It is often better to use natural substitutes that have colors resembling whatever it is they are filling in for.

A sneaky way to avoid this dilemma is to use colored containers to create an illusion of color—for example, rose-colored or lilac-colored glass. However, upon opening and examining contents, consumers might become irate. People's expectations of a product can't be understated in importance. When people don't get what they expect, they often get upset.

Packaging is very important, especially in determining sales. If you take the time to make your scented products, don't forget to package them appropriately. If packages look eloquent, they will reap more money in the marketplace than if they look crude. People expect to pay a lower price for things that look cheap.

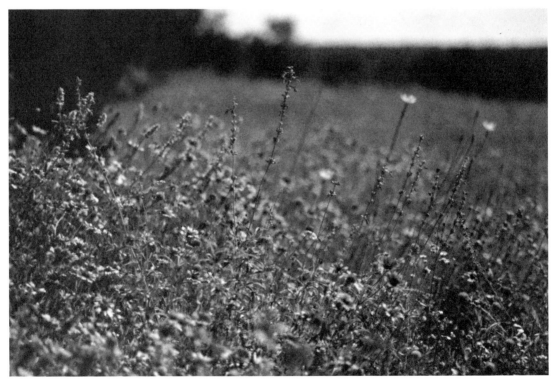

Always obtain permission from the landowner before you pick wildflowers.

SEARCHING OUT NATURE

If you don't grow flowers in your own garden, don't despair. Chances are the flowers you desire can be found within your own community. Sometimes flowers grow wild in the woods and are free for the picking. It's a good idea, however, to be sure that the flowers you pick don't belong to any protected species. To pick such flowers is against the law. If you pick flowers in an area woods, be sure to obtain permission from the owner first. Not all woodland is public property, and people often don't appreciate trespassers. Would you?

Never pick flowers found in public parks or arboretums. It is usually safe to assume those flowers are there for exhibition.

Neighbors might be willing to give, trade, or sell you the flowers and herbs that you want. However, always ask your neighbors before picking their flowers: Never assume that they don't care. Even close friendships can become strained for want of communication. Nobody likes to be taken for granted, so always show common courtesy.

Once you have obtained the flowers or herbs that you want, you'll need to dry them. Flowers can rot if they're not dried properly. Silica gel can help you achieve professional results.

Other Sources

Don't overlook your florist as a source for flowers. Although it might be more expensive, most potpourris do not require a large number of flowers. Sometimes a florist can even place a special order for you so you can obtain flowers not native to your area. Exotic flowers such as, orchids, gardenias, oleander, heliotrope, and jasmine are some examples.

By using essential oils you can obtain the fragrances that you want without using the original flower. Because these floral and herbal oils are concentrated, they are more potent than the real thing. It is important to use them *gingerly* in your potpourris. If you add too much you risk overpowering the mix and upsetting the bouquet of your potpourri. You only need one or two drops of these essential oils. A good potpourri allows you to detect a subtlety of fragrances as well as the dominant theme.

One advantage of using floral oils is that you can substitute cheaper flowers for the original. For example, dandelions—which are free for the picking—are an excellent substitute for carnations. You can even dye flowers before drying them if you want a certain color. However, avoid picking dandelions on lawns treated with herbicides. Those flowers might poison your potpourri, cause off-odors, and release poison fumes. To color your dandelions see chapter 9 for herbal colorants. Beet juice is an excellent natural dye.

Finally, many exotic flowers are often grown as houseplants. If you don't grow any yourself, check with some of your relatives and friends. You might be surprised at how easy it is to obtain a slip of a plant for you to grow on your own.

Part 2

Homemade Potpourris & Sachets

Chapter 3

English Potpourri

EACH SPRING, millions of visitors from around the world delight in the Chelsea Flower Show. It is often said that there are three things the English love: High tea (afternoon tea served at 4 p.m.), sweets, and gardening. Indeed, English gardens are the standard of the horticultural world.

Although potpourri was invented in France, it has been enjoyed as an English craft for hundreds of years. Two favorite flowers of Olden England are still grown today. These are the Red Rose of Lancaster, and the White Rose of York. These flowers have an interesting history. The Red Rose of Lancaster, (*Rosa gallica officianalis*) is actually one of the oldest roses in cultivation, predating England. One of its ancestors was used as a religious symbol of the Persians and Medes over 3,000 years ago. In England, this flower dates back to the early Middle Ages. It was brought to England by Crusaders returning home from Damascus.

The Red Rose of Lancaster is ideal for making potpourri. Its petals retain their heavenly perfume even when dried. Powdered rose petals were once used by Monks in cooking, and are still used today in conserves.

The White Rose of York, (*Rosa alba*) also dates back to the Middle Ages. It bears large white flowers that produce a heady perfume. It is one of the variety of roses grown in Eastern Europe to produce attar of roses.

Students of English history are perhaps more familiar with these roses because of their use as symbols of the opposing factions of the civil unrest known as the War of the Roses.

Horticulturists, however, are not interested in military symbols. These roses are easy to grow and can be obtained through some mail order nurseries.

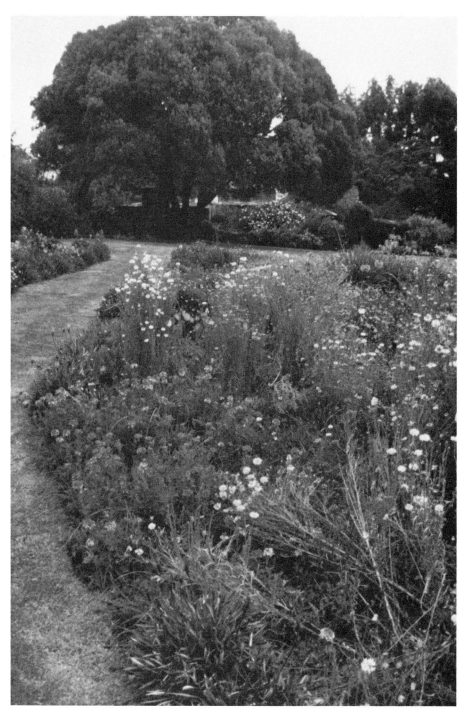

English gardens are the standard of the horticulture world.

RED ROSE OF LANCASTER POTPOURRI

1 quart dried rose petals of the Red Rose of Lancaster
3 tablespoons salt
1 ounce powdered benzoin gum
1 tablespoon deer's tongue herb
1 teaspoon nutmeg
2 teaspoons cinnamon
1 tablespoon thyme
1 drop oil of bergamot

Mix potpourri ingredients so that they are well dispersed. Cover tightly and let set overnight. Stir again in the morning, and pour into potpourri containers. You could place the potpourri in permanent containers right away; however, letting the ingredients settle tends to season it into a better potpourri.

WHITE ROSE OF YORK POTPOURRI

1 1/2 pints dried White Rose of York petals
1/2 teaspoon powdered myrrh gum
2 tablespoons salt
3 tablespoons rosemary
1 tablespoon rue
1 teaspoon vanilla
1 ounce powdered benzoin gum
1 teaspoon cinnamon
1 teaspoon allspice

ENGLISH ROSE CONSERVES

Conserves are jams made from a mixture of fruits and sometimes nuts. In Old England, powdered rose petals were also used. It is important not to use petals from flowers that have been treated with insecticides, fungicides, or herbicides, or, the conserves won't be safe to eat.

When making conserves it is important to realize that *pectin* is the "jellifying" substance. Apples contain pectin naturally. The following are two recipes for rose conserves:

RED ROSE OF LANCASTER CONSERVES

1 quart chopped Sops of Wine apples
1 pint powdered petals of the Red Rose of Lancaster
1/4 cup chopped English Walnuts
2 teaspoons grated lemon peel
1 teaspoon cinnamon

Cook for 25 minutes using the open kettle method of canning. Stir with a long-handled wooden spoon. Pour the boiling mixture into sterile jars, and place lids and rings on the jars. Use a cloth to screw covers on tightly so you don't burn yourself. Set jars aside to let them seal. Recipe makes 3 pints or 6 half-pints.

MODERN ROSE CONSERVE

2 quarts chopped tart apples (winesap, MacIntosh or Sops of Wine)
1 pint red raspberries
1/4 cup chopped English Walnuts
3 1/2 cups sugar
1 pint powdered rose petals of fragrant variety (Oklahoma, Mr. Lincoln)
1 teaspoon cinnamon
2 tablespoons lemon juice
1 package fruit pectin

Follow the cooking instructions for jams on your package of fruit pectin. You can substitute fresh rose petals for powdered rose petals, use a fragrant variety of your preferred color for best results. Use only flowers not treated with pesticides. Recipe makes approximately 9 cups.

The Ballads of Robin Hood

One of the more fascinating aspects of any nation can be found in its legends and folklore. These tales are handed down from generation to generation, some orally, others in written form.

The Ballad of Robin Hood is legend. Actually there are about forty such ballads, of which eight are of primary literary significance—and, of course, there are modern versions of this famous story.

Some evidence suggests that the original ballads were based on a true tale, but how much is true and what is fiction has never been accurately determined.

Robin Hood was a heroic figure. Although always described as a robber, he was endowed with a chivalrous and generous nature. He lived by poaching in the King's preserves in Sherwood Forest (Barnsdale Forest is also mentioned in some of the ballads). According to legend he stole only from the rich and gave to the poor, which distinguished him from the cutthroat highwaymen of his day, in that Robin Hood only stole excess wealth. Even the rich were never robbed of all their belongings and made destitute. Also, he always offered assistance to any honest person in distress.

When most people hear the name Robin Hood, they envision images of Errol Flynn or one of the other Hollywood actors who played the role in films. However, the English Ballads are more poetic and really should be read for a deeper appreciation of Old England and the legend that is Robin Hood.

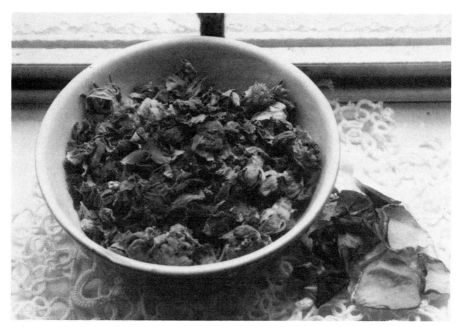

Red Rose of Lancaster potpourri.

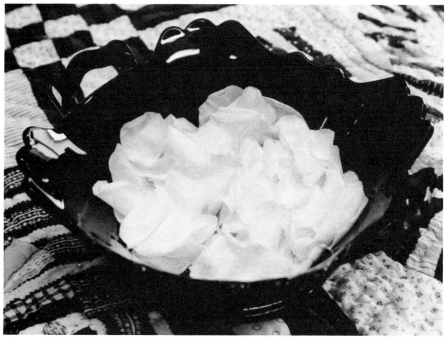

White Rose of York petals.

OLD ENGLISH POTPOURRI RECIPES

RUE AND ROSEMARY POTPOURRI

8 ounces rue (also called German Rue)
8 ounces rosemary
1 ounce powdered myrrh gum (fixative)
2 tablespoons English lavender flowers
1 vanilla bean
3 ounces deer's tongue herb
4 cloves
2 drops bergamot oil

Myrrh gum acts as a fixing agent as well as adding a perfume of its own.

SHERWOOD FOREST POTPOURRI

1 pint violet blossoms
8 ounces sweet woodruff
4 ounces thyme
4 ounces rosemary
1 ounce powdered orris root
2 ounces geranium leaves (Rober's lemon rose)
1/2 stick cinnamon (broken)
2 drops bergamot oil

ROBIN HOOD POTPOURRI

1 pint rose petals
1 tablespoon sweet woodruff
2 tablespoons dried strawberries
1 tablespoon salt
1 ounce powdered myrrh gum
1 teaspoon vanilla
2 teaspoons cinnamon

MAID MARION POTPOURRI

1 pint red rose blossoms
1/2 pint white rose petals
3 tablespoons damiana
1 ounce dried hawthorne berries
1 ounce powdered orris root
1 tablespoon lavender flowers

In 1603 James IV of Scotland became James I, King of England. His reign is probably best remembered for the Hampton Court Conference of 1604, which resulted in the decision to make the translation of the Bible, known as the King James Version. This poetic work has been a standard

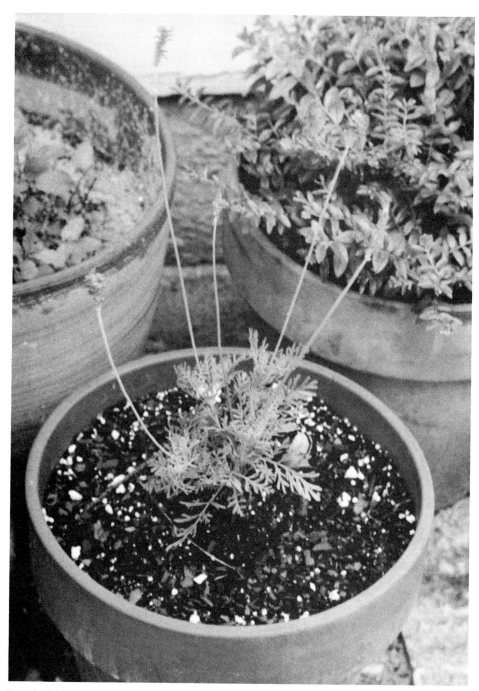

English lavender can be grown indoors or outdoors in pots.

in many Protestant congregations, although newer revisions are now replacing it. Unfortunately, many of the newer revisions have lost much of the poetic beauty that is found only in the King James Version.

King James also did something that is of particular interest to the horticultural world: He ordered the mass plantings of mulberry trees.

KING JAMES POTPOURRI

1 pint English mulberries
2 ounces rue
2 ounces rosemary
2 ounces thyme
1 ounce powdered myrrh gum
1 vanilla bean
1 ounce lemon peel

Scotland, land of clans and kilts, firths and lochs—if you close your eyes you can almost hear the din of bagpipes echoing in the Scottish Highlands.

If you ever travel to Scotland you will discover that they are a proud people. They should be addressed as "Scots," not "Scotch," which is an alcoholic beverage.

SCOTTISH HIGHLAND POTPOURRI

1 pint heather
2 ounces calendula flowers (marigolds)
1 tablespoon salt
1 ounce deer's tongue herb
1 ounce damiana
1 ounce powdered orris root
4 ounces violets

1789 ushered in a new era in England. The literature of the day dubbed it the Romantic Age. Even today just the mention of the literari of that time conjures up images of some of the great writers in the English language: William Wordsworth, Samuel Taylor Coleridge, Sir Walter Scott, Charles Lamb, and perhaps the most famous trio of all—Lord Byron, Percy Bysshe Shelley, and John Keats. Their poetry can still stir the soul, even after all this time.

The romantics subordinated reason to intuition and passion. They emphasized the supremacy of individual will over contemporary norms of social behavior.

Flowers, which were once mere articles of commerce, took on new meanings. Greek temples began appearing in parks, even though England was a Christian nation. And potpourri reflected the mood of the times.

ENGLISH ROMANCE POTPOURRI

1 pint rosebuds and petals
4 ounces lavender flowers
2 ounces sweet fern
4 ounces strawberries
1 ounce powdered orris root
1 vanilla bean

VICTORIAN AGE

Potpourri and sachet were exceedingly popular during Victorian England. This was the golden age of the British Empire: England had reached its pinnacle and would never again hold such power over the rest of the world.

Many fancy sachet pillows covered with lace could be found in the parlor of the fashionable Lord and Lady. Conservatories and windowsill gardens provided many of the plants used for making potpourris. New and exotic plants came in from the far reaches of the British Empire, offering a wide assortment of floral delights to the English gentry.

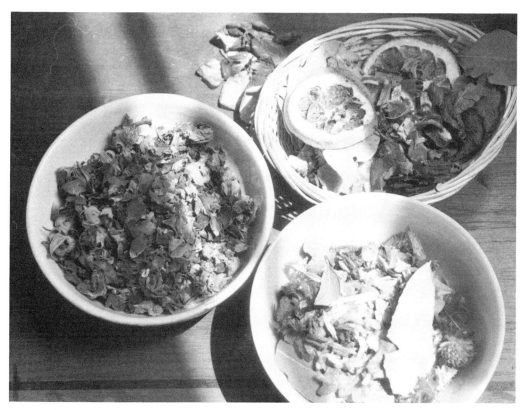

Potpourri was an English craft for hundreds of years.

VANILLA POTPOURRI

1 pint White Rose of York petals
2 ounces rosemary
2 ounces rue
1 ounce myrrh gum
1 cinnamon stick
2 vanilla beans
1 ounce lemon peel

VICTORIAN LAVENDER SACHET

8 ounces corn or potato starch
4 ounces talc or chalk powder
1 ounce powdered orris root
1 ounce lavender flowers
1 teaspoon vanilla
1 drop bergamot oil

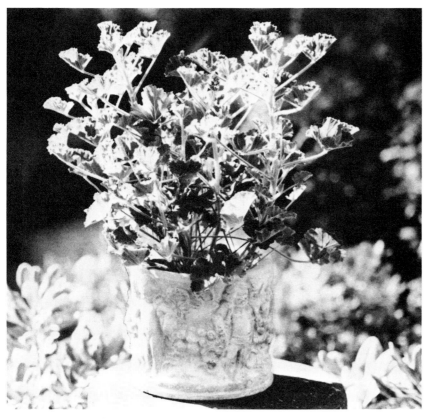

Lemon-scented geraniums.

COUNTESS OF SCARBOROUGH POTPOURRI

1 pint rosebuds and petals
4 ounces geranium leaves (Countess of Scarborough variety, strawberry-scented)
2 ounces rosemary
2 ounces juniper berries
1 ounce myrrh gum (powdered)
1 teaspoon cinnamon
1 vanilla bean
1 drop bergamot oil

Regional Recipes

CANTERBURY POTPOURRI

1/4 pint calendula flowers (marigolds)
1/2 pint canterbury bells
1 ounce rosemary
1 ounce juniper berries
2 ounces geranium leaves (nutmeg variety)
1 ounce powdered balsam of Peru (fixative)

BATH POTPOURRI

2 ounces geranium leaves (parviflorum species, coconut-scented)
2 ounces sweet fern
1 ounce deer's tongue herb
1 ounce lavender flowers
1 ounce powdered myrrh gum
2 drops almond oil

WHITE CLIFFS OF DOVER POTPOURRI

1 pint White Rose of York petals
2 ounces chalk powder
1 ounce powdered benzoin gum
1 vanilla bean
2 drops bergamot oil

PENZANCE POTPOURRI

1 tablespoon orange peel
1 ounce shredded coconut
1 ounce English spearmint
1 cinnamon stick
1 vanilla bean
1 ounce powdered benzoin gum
1 tablespoon lemon peel

STRATFORD-ON-AVON POTPOURRI

2 ounces parsley
2 ounces sage
2 ounces rosemary (pine-scented rosemary, *angustifolis*)
2 ounces thyme
1 ounce juniper berries
1 ounce deer's tongue herb
1 ounce violets
1 ounce powdered orris root
1 drop bergamot oil

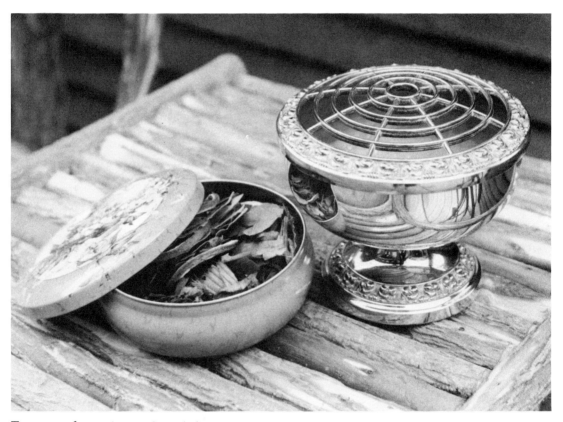

Two popular potpourri containers.

Chapter 4

Other European Potpourris

EUROPE. Even the name conjures up images of castles and palaces, stone cottages, and Alpine chalets. Europe is a land of many contrasts. Some of the contrasts are obvious, such as the clatter of horsehooves on cobblestone streets and the din of the fast-paced traffic on the Autobahn. In Europe, the very old and the very new converge.

Europe is comprised of many nations and even more diverse ethnic groups between and within each nation. The dominant powers on the continent are Germany, France, Italy and Russia. However, because the Soviet Union's society has been a closed one for many years, its cultural influence has been severely restricted.

The European nations have had a tremendous influence on the West. France has been especially pivotal in the English-speaking world. With the unification of western Europe in the near future, there can be no doubt that Europe and its people will continue to influence and perhaps set the pace for much of humanity.

FRENCH POTPOURRIS

France, world famous for its perfumes, is also credited with the invention of potpourri. France is the birthplace of the modern hybrid tea rose.

Perhaps the most famous hybrid tea rose is Peace. It was named the day that Berlin fell during the second world war. The Peace rose was developed by renowned rose breeder, Francis Meilland.

Hybrid teas are by far the most popular of the rose family, understandably so because of their grace of form. Some are also quite fragrant. However, many of the older variety and species roses have richer fragrance and are preferrable for potpourris, colognes, and perfumes.

One class of aromatic roses are the Bourbon hybrids. Many of these are descended from roses grown in the famous garden of the Empress Josephine at Malmaison. Bourbon hybrids are progenitors to many modern types.

Some of the best *culivars* (cultivated varieties) for aromatic essence are:

- ❀ **Madame Isaac Pereire** has dark crimson blossoms with a rich, fruity, raspberry perfume. It is one of the most fragrant roses.
- ❀ **Souvenir de la Malmaison** has pale pink blooms and is very fragrant.
- ❀ **Louise Odier** has deep pink blossoms and produces a heady perfume.

It is very important to note that different roses have different aromatic essences, so to obtain the truest quality, recipes should not substitute one type of rose for another. The following recipes are inspired by the ancient regime.

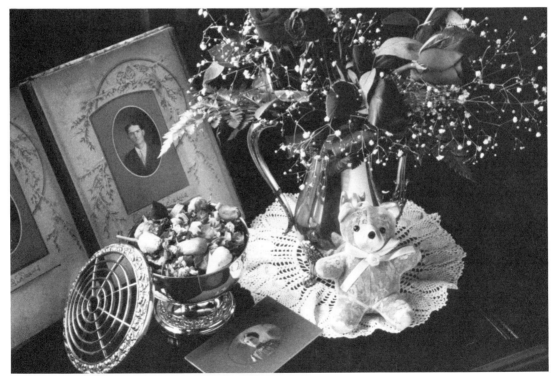

Rose potpourri is a favorite in Europe.

OLD FRENCH POTPOURRI RECIPES

EMPRESS JOSEPHINE POTPOURRI

1 pint Souvenir de la Malmaison petals and rosebuds
2 tablespoons brown sugar
1 ounce sweet bay
1 ounce powdered orris root
4 ounces violets (parma violets)
2 ounces white bonnet (feverfew flowers)
3 tablespoons raspberry brandy

Stir potpourri so that the ingredients are well dispersed. Let set in a covered container overnight. Stir again in the morning, and pour into potpourri containers. The reason for letting the mixture set overnight is so that the various aromatic essences settle, resulting in a richer perfume.

KING CHARLES X POTPOURRI

1 pint Madame Isaac Pereire rosebuds and petals
1 ounce parma violets
2 ounces geranium leaves (French Lace)
1 tablespoon salt
1 vanilla bean
1 ounce powdered frankincense (fixative)

DUKE OF ORLEANS POTPOURRI

1 pint violets
1 tablespoon salt
1 teaspoon nutmeg
1 ounce powdered orris root
1 cinnamon stick (broken)
1 ounce cognac
4 ounces white bonnet (feverfew flowers)
1 teaspoon vanilla

JARDINS DE BAGATELLE POTPOURRI

1/4 pint Madame Isaac Pereire rosebuds
1/4 pint Louise Odier rosebuds
2 ounces white bonnet (feverfew flowers)
2 ounces violets (parma)
1 ounce powdered myrrh gum (fixative)
1 vanilla bean
1 drop bergamot oil

In the valleys of southern France, jasmine flowers have been grown for over 900 years. In the 17th century, French nobility declared jasmine as the royal fragrance of France.

ROYAL JASMINE POTPOURRI

1 pint jasmine flowers
4 ounces white bonnets (feverfew flowers)
2 ounces calendula flowers (marigolds)
1 ounce deer's tongue herb
1 ounce German rue
1 ounce powdered frankincense gum (fixative)
1 vanilla bean

Napolean

A Napolean rag doll posed with his hand in his coat is sure to be a favorite of any toddler. To scent your rag doll, sew the potpourri packet in his coat. Locate it in the same spot as the heart, or sew the packet into the center of the doll itself. One advantage of keeping it external, is that the potpourri can be "freshened" over time.

For parents concerned about the military aspect, this former emperor looks more cute and cuddly than ferocious, and it's easy to give Napolean a candy cane in lieu of a sword. It makes for a cute toy that children of all ages will enjoy for years to come.

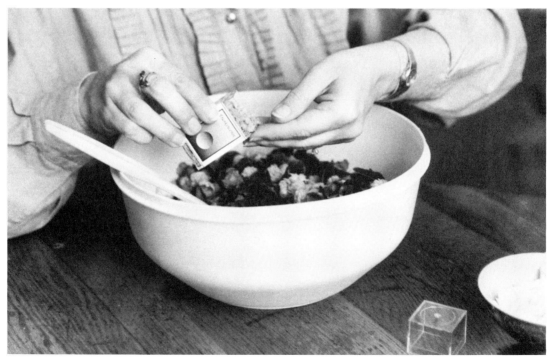

While it helps to follow recipes when you're first learning to make potpourri, you can always experiment to find your own special "blend."

NAPOLEAN'S SWORD POTPOURRI

2 ounces potato starch
1 ounce talc
1 ounce powdered benzoin gum
2 ounces peppermint (black peppermint)
1 teaspoon vanilla
1 drop oil of bergamot

NAPOLEON SACHET

2 ounces cornstarch
1 ounce talc
1 ounce peppermint (black peppermint)
1 ounce violets
1 ounce jasmine blossoms
1 ounce powdered frankincense (fixative)
1 teaspoon vanilla

GERMAN POTPOURRIS

Germans rank second only to the English in terms of their emigration to the United States during its formative years, so it is only natural that Germany holds a special fascination to Americans, with so many of German ancestry.

Modern Germany, as the rest of Europe, is a land of many contrasts. It has both large cities and rustic villages. Castles along the Rhine River remind visitors of the rich history of the German people.

The German nation is relatively new in European politics. Germany, like Italy to its south, has existed as a group of independent principalities throughout much of its history.

A visitor to Germany can find much to see. Those interested in fragrances must see Köln, where cologne was invented. People interested in fine china can find a wide selection at Dresden. But the Black Forest might be one of the most popular haunts. Nestled in the Black Forest, German craftsmen and craftswomen produce handicrafts famous the world over.

BLACK FOREST POTPOURRI

2 ounces geranium leaves (Village Hill Oak, pine-scented)
1 ounce balsam fir needles
2 ounces German rue
4 ounces sweet woodruff
2 tablespoons pine needles
3 tablespoons cedar chips
1 ounce powdered orris root
1 tablespoon violets
1 drop bergamot oil
1 teaspoon vanilla

Hansel and Gretel

Most children round the world are familiar with the fairy tale of Hansel and Gretel, the witch, and her house made of gingerbread. A Hansel or Gretel rag doll could easily become a favorite of your toddlers. Adventuresome parents might even wish to sew a witch rag doll, or even to construct a cardboard gingerbread house to make the set complete. (See chapter 7 for Gingerbread Potpourri recipe.) If you do make a witch doll, try to make it less frightening for small children.

Several companies sell patterns that you can use to make rag dolls. Check the appendix of this book for a listing to purchase patterns, or design your own.

Just as with other rag dolls, always place the potpourri inside the doll so younger children cannot tamper with it or accidentally swallow the potpourri. Be aware of your children's allergies and don't use ingredients that might cause an allergic reaction: Use a substitute if the recipe calls for something known to you as an allergin.

Never use poisonous herbs in potpourris for children. For example, the herb known as *deer's tongue* is poisonous. It won't affect adults (unless they eat it), but children often put things into their mouths. Also, natural bergamot oil can cause allergic reactions and skin rash. Don't use this as an ingredient in potpourris your children might have access to.

HANSEL POTPOURRI

1 ounce rue
1 ounce sweet woodruff
1 tablespoon cedar chips
1 tablespoon rosemary
1/2 ounce powdered orris root
1 teaspoon lemon peel
1 teaspoon vanilla
1/4 teaspoon ginger
1 ounce peppermint (black peppermint)

GRETEL POTPOURRI

1 ounce rue
1 ounce sweet woodruff
1 ounce violets
1 tablespoon rosebuds and petals
1 tablespoon rosemary
1/2 ounce powdered orris root
1 teaspoon vanilla
1 teaspoon lemon peel
1/4 teaspoon ginger
1 ounce peppermint (black peppermint)

WITCH'S POTPOURRI

2 ounces witchhazel
1 ounce rosemary
1 ounce rue
1 ounce powdered myrrh gum
1 ounce sweet woodruff
1 teaspoon lemon peel
1/4 teaspoon ginger
2 teaspoons vanilla

PEPPERMINT CANDY CANE POTPOURRI

4 ounces rosebuds and petals
2 ounces peppermint (black peppermint)
1 ounce powdered orris root
1 tablespoon lemon peel
1 teaspoon cinnamon

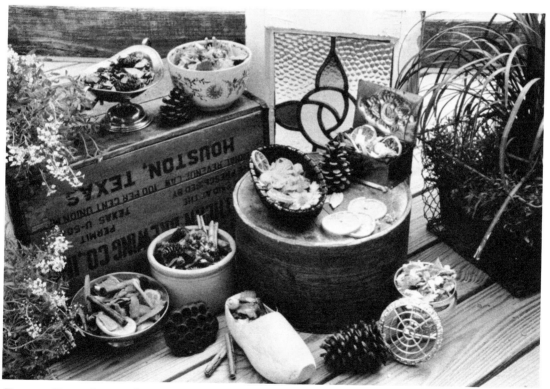

Be creative when selecting a potpourri container.

ITALIAN POTPOURRIS

Italy is a land of culture and romance. The ancient city of Rome was once capital of a great empire that stretched from Britain in the north to Carthage in the south. Many splendid ruins from Rome's past remain intact, such as the Coloseum.

If you are looking for culture, the city of Florence is the place to see paintings and works of sculpture by Italian masters from the past. Don't forget to take the train to Venice to see the canals and the city where Marco Polo once lived.

The modern Italian nation is also relatively new to European politics. Italy, like its German neighbor spent much of its history as a collection of principalities. Of course it was united during the Roman Empire, and for a few brief times in between. Italy was a kingdom prior to 1946.

Pinocchio

One of the best-loved Italian folktales is that of Gepetto and his wooden marionette (puppet), Pinocchio. According to the story, Pinocchio's nose would grow every time he told a lie. This was a fairy tale with a happy ending as Pinocchio becomes a real boy, fulfilling both his wishes and the dream of Gepetto, who carved him from wood.

A Pinocchio doll always pleases the youngsters. Ambitious parents might enjoy making a Gepetto rag doll as well. Commercial patterns are available, or you might prefer using your own designs.

PINOCCHIO POTPOURRI

2 ounces cedar chips
1 ounce sweet woodruff
1 ounce rue
1 ounce powdered sandalwood (fixative)
1 teaspoon nutmeg
1 teaspoon vanilla

GEPETTO POTPOURRI

2 ounces savory
1 ounce Italian oregano
1 ounce sweet bay
2 tablespoons lemon balm
1 tonka bean
1 ounce powdered frankincense (fixative)
1/4 teaspoon cinnamon

Chapter 5

Oriental Potpourri

SINCE THE DAYS of Marco Polo, the Orient has held a special fascination for European peoples and people of the Occident (west). Many European merchants became wealthy off the spice trade. People would pay dearly to obtain the wondrous spices of the Orient, which added zest to often bland fare. Later, many of these same spices were used for their fragrances in potpourris.

Exotic flowers brought from the Orient helped breathe new life into the horticultural world as new hybrids were born. Perhaps the most famous example is the hybrid tea rose of today: Its progenitors came from China.

Although Asia covers many countries and cultures, three pivotal societies are India, China, and Japan

INDIAN POTPOURRI

When Columbus discovered the Americas it was by accident. He was en route to India. Columbus believed the Earth was round, so he thought by going West he'd end up in the East. His expedition was hoping to find a shortcut to India, as the treasures of India were well-known. Columbus was right, but he hadn't realized the world was as big as it is, so he ended up in the New World.

Thinking at first that he had reached India, Columbus called the natives that he encountered "Indians." This misnomer has stuck with them to this day. Of the multitude of tribes of Native Americans, all are commonly called "Indians," although none of them are of Indo-Aryan origin.

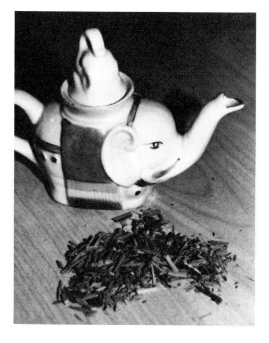

Sandalwood is a favorite Indian scent.

The New India

Today, India is a rapidly developing nation. Prior to Britain's long and often inhumane occupation, India existed as a collection of principalities, much like Medieval Italy and Germany.

After great sacrifice, India achieved its independence from the United Kingdom. The nations of Pakistan and Bangladesh were also once part of the British Mandate. Today, they are independent nations with predominantly Moslem populations, although smaller religious sects exist in all three nations.

BOMBAY POTPOURRI

4 ounces patchouli leaves
1 ounce powdered frankincense (fixative)
2 ounces sandalwood shavings
1 cinnamon stick
1 tonka bean

Taj Mahal

The most beautiful building in the world is one way to describe the Taj Mahal. Located in Agra, it was built by order of the Mogul Emperor of Hindustan, Shah Jahan. It is actually a mausoleum of white marble and alabaster. It was erected as a burial place for Shah Jahan's favorite wife, Mumtaz Mahal, who died in 1631.

The Taj Mahal was designed by an architect named, Ustad Isa. It was constructed between 1632-1650 A.D. The building consists of a square structure of white marble. The dome rises to a height of 210 feet. The bodies of Shah Jahan and his wife, Mumtaz Mahal, are buried in the vault beneath the central chamber. Above them are alabaster screens inlaid with precious stones.

Daylight filters through the perforated alabaster screens of the windows and translucent alabaster of the dome. The exterior is decorated with passages from the Koran (Islam's holy book).

The building sets upon a terrace on a hill. At the corners stand four cylinder *minerets* (prayer towers), each 133 feet tall. A rectangular pond lies in front of the Taj Mahal. Also, at the front is a gateway with two mosques (temples) built of red sandstone and white marble.

The gardens of the Taj Mahal are home to many beautiful and aromatic flowers.

TAJ MAHAL POTPOURRI

1 pint heliotrope blossoms
4 ounces garden pinks (Fair Folley Dianthus)
2 ounces oleander blossoms
1 ounce powdered myrrh gum (fixative)
4 ounces patchouli leaves
1 tonka bean

CALCUTTA POTPOURRI

4 ounces khus khus
4 ounces patchouli leaves
4 ounces sandalwood chips (fixative)
2 ounces heliotrope flowers
1 nutmeg
1 cinnamon stick
1 tonka bean

Sri Lanka

Sri Lanka, formerly known as Ceylon, is a small island nation off the coast of southern India.

SRI LANKA POTPOURRI

2 ounces khus khus (vetiver)
1 ounce orange pekoe tea
1 ounce patchouli leaves
1 stick cinnamon
1 ounce heliotrope
1 ounce lemon peel
1 ounce powdered sandalwood (fixative)

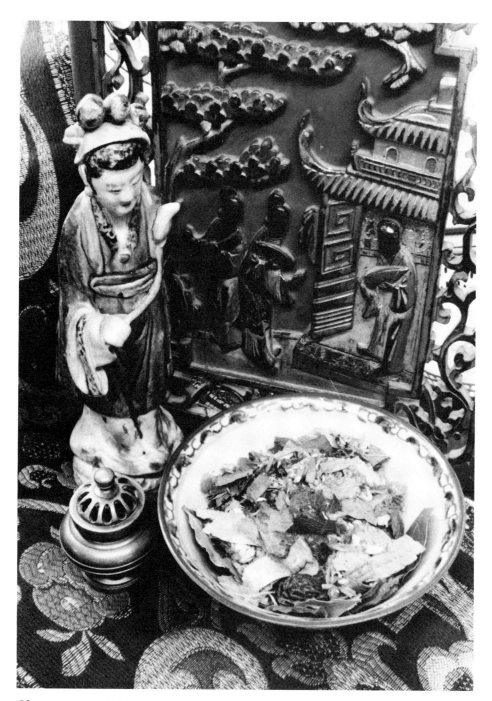

Chinese potpourri.

CHINESE POTPOURRI

As one of the oldest continuous societies, China is extremely fascinating. It is also one of the oldest civilizations in the world, offering a wealth of history and knowledge. The flora (plant life) is of special interest to horticulturists and botanists.

Many species of roses are found in China. Roses have been cultivated in China since ancient times when they were grown in the lavish gardens of royal families. Horticulturally, the most important rose to come out of China is the tea rose, *Rose odorata*. The tea rose was crossed with European roses in France to create the famous hybrid tea roses of today.

CHINA ROSE POTPOURRI

1 pint China Rose petals
4 ounces oleander blossoms
1 ounce powdered myrrh gum (fixative)
1 vanilla bean

CATHAY ROSE POTPOURRI

1 pint Cathay Rosebuds and petals
1 tonka bean
1 stick cinnamon
1 ounce quassia chips
1 ounce powdered orris root

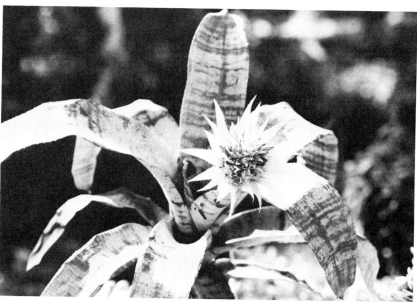

Exotic flowers can be grown in pots.

YUANMINGYUAN GARDENS POTPOURRI

1 pint wisteria blossoms
2 ounces oleander blossoms
2 ounces heliotrope flowers
4 ounces ylang ylang blossoms
2 ounces tea rosebuds
1 ounce frankincense gum
1 teaspoon vanilla
1/4 teaspoon cinnamon

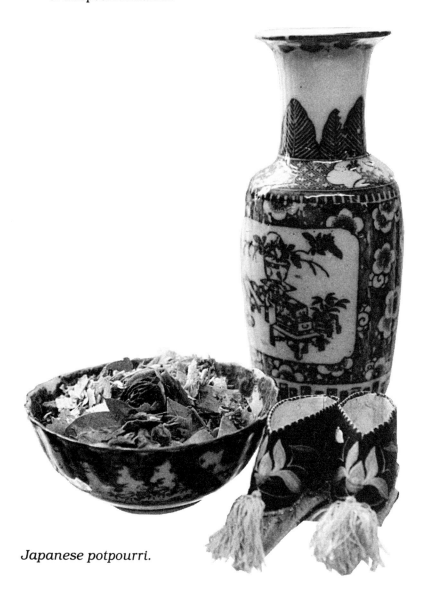

Japanese potpourri.

CHINESE TEA ROSE POTPOURRI

1 pint Chinese Tea Rosebuds and petals
4 ounces wisteria blossoms
1 ounce powdered frankincense (fixative)
2 ounces oleander blossoms
1 teaspoon cinnamon bark

XI'AN POTPOURRI

1 pint wisteria blossoms
4 ounces China Rosebuds
1 ounce powdered myrrh gum (fixative)
1 tablespoon lemon peel
1 teaspoon vanilla

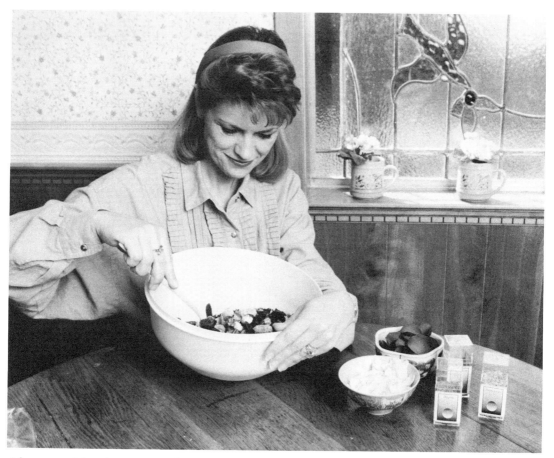

Always add spices gingerly.

SHANGHAI POTPOURRI

4 ounces orange blossoms
2 ounces heliotrope flowers
2 ounces ylang ylang flowers
1 ounce frankincense (fixative)
1 teaspoon nutmeg
1 teaspoon orange peel
$^1/_2$ teaspoon cinnamon
1 teaspoon vanilla

JAPANESE POTPOURRI

Japan is known as the land of the rising sun. Over 17,000 species of flowering and nonflowering plants are found in Japan. Many exotic flowers have been brought over from Japan from which new hybrids have been developed.

JAPANESE POTPOURRI

4 ounces camellia blossoms
2 ounces rose petals
1 ounce powdered benzoin gum
1 vanilla bean
1 teaspoon pine needles

NIPPON GARDEN POTPOURRI

8 ounces chrysanthemum flowers
4 ounces carnations
2 ounces hibiscus flowers
1 tonka bean
1 ounce powdered benzoin gum
1 tablespoon orange peel
1 teaspoon allspice
1 teaspoon sandalwood
1 teaspoon oleander blossoms

Chapter 6

Americana

cAMERICAN AND CANADIAN families have for generations enjoyed the delights of homemade potpourris and sachets. Your grandmother might have a secret family recipe, or you might have a few of your own. One thing is for certain: These are home crafts that the entire family can enjoy making together.

Because of the shortage of family time together, many people set aside one night of the week when they agree to not watch television. That gives the family time to do things together that they would normally spend as couch potatoes. Perhaps such a scheme could work in your household.

NATIVE AMERICAN DREAM PILLOWS

Contrary to popular belief, the science of *aromatherapy* is not entirely new. Several American Indian Nations have long employed potpourris in their practice of natural medicine and in their traditional religious worship, much as incense is used in Eastern Churches.

The importance of fragrance and the sense of smell to physical well-being is only now being investigated by scientific researchers. Surprisingly, they are finding some validity in the old rituals.

Making a Dream Pillow

Construct a pillow by sewing a tightly-knit cloth together at three sides. Cotton is the best material to use because it breathes; many man-made fabrics do not.

Most dream pillows are not very large. These pillows will not be used to prop your head up on in the bed. They should go next to your head, or inside the pillowcase of your regular pillow. The important thing is that they be near your face at night so you can breathe the fragrances they emit. Dream pillows are said to affect your subconscious mind, causing lucid dreams.

CHEROKEE DREAM PILLOW POTPOURRI

2 ounces lavender flowers
1 ounce cedar shavings
2 ounces sage
2 ounces coltsfoot herb
1 ounce ground orris root
2 ounces sweet fern
2 ounces deer's tongue herb
1 ounce violets

OJIBWA DREAM POTPOURRI

2 ounces sweet vernal grass
2 ounces sunbul root (smells like musk)
1 ounce goldenthread root
1 ounce ground orris root
2 ounces chopped vetiver

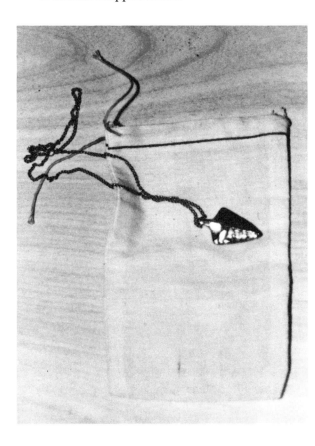

Native American Dream Pillow.

PIONEER POTPOURRI

2 ounces geranium leaves (True Rose)
2 ounces sweet woodruff
2 ounces Life Everlasting flowers
2 ounces sweet meliot
2 ounces rosemary
2 ounces sweet fern
1 ounce ground orris root
1 ounce rue

SACHET PILLOWS

Sachet pillows are an excellent use for potpourris. People usually don't use potpourri sewn in pillow form because the cloth covering hides the colors, texture, and beauty of the dried flowers, herbs, and spices. Sachets, on the other hand, have fragrance, but are more finely ground. Their powdery filling lacks the aesthetic appeal of potpourri.

All powders are somewhat similar in appearance, tending to mask their uniqueness. For example, wheat and rye flours vary somewhat in appearance, but not appreciably so—not enough to arouse interest or attention in the same way as various potpourris do.

Unless you are using a clear vinyl or cheaper plastic see-through material, your sachet pillows will most likely not depend upon content for visual appeal. Scent alone will be their function, so you might wish to make the pillows as attractive as possible with embroidery and/or lace.

You do not have to buy special cloth for your sachet projects. You can probably use the good sections of old dresses, shirts, or other items of clothing as a base. Test the cloth by pulling both ways on the fabric. Do *not* use the worn out parts of garments. (Portions close to underarms or "seats" are always suspect.)

Two other points to remember are:

❀ All materials should be clean. Never use dirty rags or musty-smelling old clothes.
❀ Undergarments are not ordinarily suited to this purpose, especially old cotton drawers. However, fancy satin or silk undergarments, if the fabric is like-new, can and do make attractive pillows.

Always use a tightly-woven fabric as an inner lining for sachet or potpourri pillows. This inner pouch will hold the fine powders in, protecting the sachet or potpourri, as well as prolonging the aromatic qualities of the product.

Sachet pillows are easy to make and can take many forms, depending upon the amount of time and expertise you devote to them. More elaborate designs might require a sewing machine.

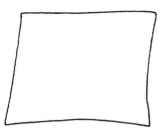

1. Take a suitable piece of cloth.

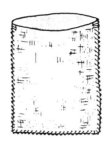
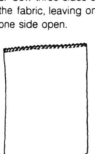

2. Sew three sides of . the fabric, leaving only one side open.

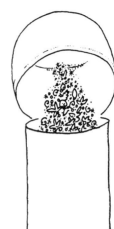

3. Turn the pillow inside out. Pour the sachet powder into the pillow until it is one-half to three-fourths full. Leave room to sew the top.

4. Sew the top of the pillow so no sachet powder can escape.

How to make a dream pillow.

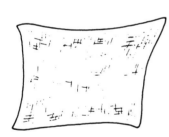

1. Take a suitable piece of cloth.

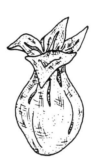

2. Fold the cloth into a little bag.

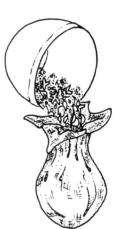

3. With one hand hold the bag. Loosen your grip and pour the sachet powder slowly into the bag until it is half full.

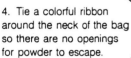
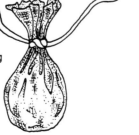

4. Tie a colorful ribbon around the neck of the bag so there are no openings for powder to escape.

5. Tie the ribbon into a bow for an attractive touch.

How to make sachets.

Extra care is needed at the beginning stage. Before you begin, select the design you want and make a pattern. Make sure the pattern is accurate because a sloppy pattern can result in a sloppy finished product. Remember also to allow room in your patterns for the natural shrinkage that occurs in the sewing process—that is, the inches lost in seam allowances. If you are using a fabric that might shrink when washed, wash it *before* you begin sewing so that it is the size you want. When you need to wash material before sewing, you'll also need to iron it. Obviously, don't use a hotter iron than your fabric will tolerate.

The inner pouch doesn't have to be as attractive as the exterior of the pillow, as it will likely never be seen. However, it still should consist of a clean, tightly-woven material. Muslin cotton, or some cotton blend is preferable to synthetic fabrics because such fabrics allow the product to breath. This is extremely important as potpourri or sachet need to be able to cross the boundaries of the covering fabric, or its aroma will be trapped and not available to enjoy.

Size is another factor that you'll want to consider in advance. How big or how little should your pillows be? That depends on several things, including the purpose you have in mind for your finished products. For the most part, small pillows will be desired. You will most likely want to make several small pillows rather than one large one. Financial considerations might be involved: Potpourri and sachet powders are somewhat costly to make. Also, these pillows have potent fragrances, so a huge pillow might be too strongly scented to enjoy.

If you want to make extra-large pillows, instead of stuffing them with potpourri or sachet powder, you might simply sew small pockets of potpourri or sachet powder into the inner lining, then use some other bulky filler for stuffing. That way you can create large, full-size pillows that are lightly scented and practical. Keep the sachet-filled pouch close to the surface, or you might inadvertently "lose" the scent altogether or weaken it too drastically.

If you have some expertise at the sewing machine or have friends who do, you might want to create special items, such as scented dolls (rag dolls) or even scented doilies.

To create a scented doily, you need only have a center pocket into which you can slip the sachet powder. Try to make the pocket thin so that it doesn't lump when the doily is spread out. Powders work best for doilies, unless you have a special design—a duck, for instance—in the center. The duck, dove, or swan, or whatever can be filled with the aromatic blend. Projects of this type require more skill than adding a hidden pocket to the underside of an already existing doily.

Sachet Recipes

AMERICAN ROSE SACHET

2 ounces cornstarch
1 ounce talc
$1/2$ ounce powdered orris root
2 drops rose oil
$1/4$ teaspoon cinnamon

ENGLISH LAVENDER SACHET

2 ounces cornstarch
1 ounce talc
$1/2$ ounce powdered orris root
1 drop lavender oil
1 drop bergamot oil

WILDFLOWER SACHET

2 ounces potato starch
1 ounce talc
$1/2$ ounce powdered benzoin gum
$1/4$ ounce sweet woodruff
$1/4$ ounce heather
1 teaspoon vanilla
1 drop violet oil

SACHET ON A ROPE

Sachet pillows secured to a rope of brightly-colored yarn makes an attractive, aromatic display. Sachet on a rope can be used to hang around doorways to thwart unpleasant odors, as in bathrooms or kitchens.

These rope sachets are relatively easy to make. The "rope" is best made from yarn, although you could braid rags or use other materials as well. The sachet pillows should be quite tiny. Alternate a number of them along the rope, leaving empty spaces in between: You won't want to over-power the area with fragrance. For a clever change of pace, try alternating fragrances to create an interesting bouquet, but be sure to avoid fragrances that clash. For example, rose and ylang ylang or peppermint and lilac fragrances don't blend well. It is usually best to stick with a central theme for each rope and have the sachets follow that general idea.

With most sachets on a rope, a hanger is added at the top for ease in displaying. Here again, you can follow a standard design or create your own.

One sachet pillow every four inches apart on a two foot rope is the standard practice, but you can vary it as you like.

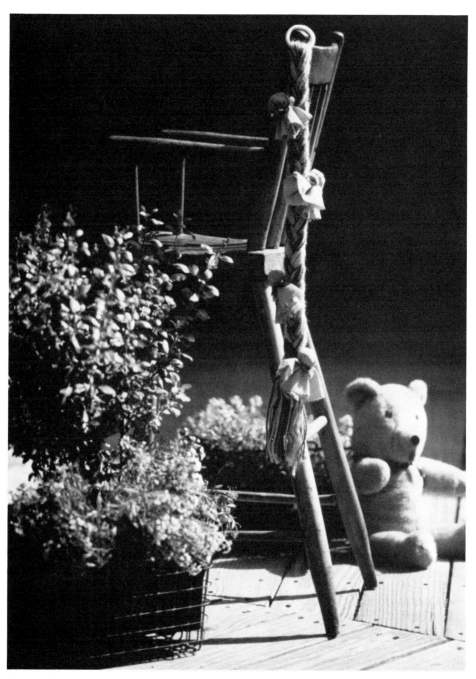

Sachet on a rope.

SACHETS FOR PACKAGES AND LETTERS

If you want to perfume your packages, add tiny sachet pillows to the package lining.

Letters can be perfumed by dusting the stationery with sachet powder or cologne. Powder often works best because it won't leave marks the way that liquid does. Also, it won't cause the ink to run or interfere with the contents of the letter, as liquids can.

When dusting a letter, do so after it has been written. If you dust the paper before you write, it can make it harder to write on the paper because some of the sachet powder will cling to the paper. If you dust after writing, you won't have that problem.

When dusting letters with powder, use a light hand. Blow off excess powder. You only need a tiny amount to perfume the letter. Any excess powder will accumulate as the letter travels. You don't want the recipient to open the letter and have a lot of sachet powder falling all over him or her. You just want them to enjoy the perfume and think of you each time they read the letter or sniff the envelope.

Sachet pillows are most practical for packages. Place the pillows in strategic locations throughout the package. It is usually not desirable to dust contents in packages.

Use your imagination when using sachet powders to perfume stationery and packages. A certain scent can be your "hallmark" to a friend or sweetheart. A special occasion or holiday may provide a clue for a theme. For example, cinnamon and other spices make excellent themes for Thanksgiving or Christmas holidays. Children are especially fond of peppermint scents. If you want a more religious expression, use frankincense and myrrh as the central theme.

SWEETHEART DOLL

Sachets and potpourri can be used to perfume your favorite rag doll. Little Judy's favorite doll can have a "potpourri heart." Think of the joyful expression on your daughter's or granddaughter's face when you give this fragrant beauty to her. She'll know it's really something special because you made it yourself!

How about making a boy rag doll for your toddler son or grandson? Boys need to learn nurturing too, or they might never grow up to be loving fathers and family-oriented men. What a delightful way to learn; through child's play!

How To Make A Sweetheart Doll

Sew a rag doll from a pattern or your own design. If you are short on time you can buy a rag doll. To make it into a sweetheart doll you will need to sew on the sachet heart.

If you are making the rag doll from scratch, you might choose to place the sachet pillow inside the doll, but don't bury it too deeply: Remember, you want the fragrance to come through. A tiny sachet pouch should be placed within a heart-shape sachet pillow. Red satin trimmed with lace is most popular, but don't be afraid to use other fabrics and colors too.

You might have the child pick out the fabric or color, but it is usually best to offer some guidance to young children. They might not be aware of symbols, such as that people expect hearts to be red. If junior insists on a black heart, try to encourage the little sweetie to choose red instead. It's all right to be unconventional, but neighbors will talk if something strikes them as weird!

Your boy will probably feel more at ease if his sweetheart doll is a boy rag doll and isn't dressed too frilly. Some people like to have their dolls dressed in various uniforms such as those of a postman, fireman, or baseball player. You might want to stay clear of policeman, pirate, or soldier uniforms; they may give a different signal to the child. Remember to sew the heart-shaped sachet pillow onto the doll's chest where the heart would be in real life—that's what makes it a "sweetheart doll."

PINCUSHIONS

Many people like to make potpourri pincushions. Pincushion patterns are available commercially. See the back of this book for companies that sell patterns.

Potpourri works better than sachet for pincushions. Every time you stick a pin in the cushion you create a hole, so powder would leak out more easily than potpourri pieces would. A good rule of thumb is to use coarser pieces in the mix than you use for making regular potpourris.

ROSE PINCUSHION POTPOURRI

4 ounces rosebuds and petals
1 ounce granular frankincense (fixative)
2 ounces lavender flowers
2 ounces rosemary
1 cinnamon stick

VIOLET PINCUSHION POTPOURRI

4 ounces violet blossoms
1 ounce cut orris root
1 ounce rose petals
1 ounce cut sunbulroot

LILY-OF-THE-VALLEY PINCUSHION POTPOURRI

4 ounces lily-of-the-valley blossoms
1 ounce rose petals
1 ounce cut orris root
1 vanilla bean

POTPOURRI FOR YOUR PETS

Fido or Fluffy can also enjoy the delights of potpourri. Dogs have a keen sense of smell, as do cats. Your pets will appreciate a gift of potpourri in the form of a pillow, to freshen their favorite nesting area.

When making a potpourri pillow for pets, be sure that you make it out of durable cotton. In addition, be sure to double-sew the seams (as in jeans). Use two layers to help prevent the pillow from getting torn: Animals can be very destructive in their play. When making your potpourri, *never* add any ingredient that will arouse an animal's sense of hunger. *Never* add catnip to a potpourri for your cat. Lemon and other citrus scents work nicely. They also have the added benefit of repelling fleas.

You can also use potpourri in your kitty litter box to freshen it.

FIDO'S POTPOURRI

2 ounces sweet woodruff
1 ounce cedarwood shavings
1 ounce sandalwood shavings (fixative)
1 ounce pine needles
1 ounce lemon peel
1 vanilla bean

FLUFFY'S POTPOURRI

2 ounces sweet woodruff
1 ounce vetiver
1 ounce lemon peel
1 ounce granular benzoin gum
1 vanilla bean

Chapter 7

Christmas

CHRISTMAS is the busiest shopping season of the year. It is also a time of the year for families to come together and remember the days of "auld lang syne."

You might want to budget your time by planning a holiday schedule when creating homemade gifts. This helps to keep things going smoothly during this hectic, albeit joyous, season.

You will be able to save money by creating your own Christmas gifts. Plan family projects well in advance of Christmas so that they can be completed on time. Always allow extra time for unexpected interruptions so you'll be able to meet your deadlines. The last thing you want is to be working on your Christmas presents after Christmas!

Make Christmas extra special in your home by planning projects in which the entire family can participate. And take time to laugh together, for it is "the season to be jolly."

OH, TANNENBAUM!

All over the world Christians celebrate the birth of the Christ child. It is a special time when family and friends gather together in time-honored rituals.

"Oh Tannenbaum!," chimes the famous German Christmas Carol. It is from this European tradition that the Christmas tree was introduced and has remained a major part of the contemporary celebration in much of the world. To many people, it just wouldn't seem like Christmas without the traditional Christmas tree. Coniferous trees, such as pine and fir, are most often used as Christmas trees. In some countries, such as Australia, eucalyptus trees are used as a substitute.

Most people prefer the traditional coniferous tree. Today there are many types of trees to choose from, including artificial trees made from plastic, metal, cloth, or paper. Some people object to the idea of growing a tree only to cut it down for one brief Christmas season. Some use artificial trees for the economy of them, as they can be dismantled and used time and again. If kept in good condition, artificial trees can last through several Christmases, although they rarely last a lifetime. Parts get lost, branches get bent, and time takes its toll.

Some people prefer real trees. One big advantage is that real trees have a fragrance that plastic trees do not. Whatever your family preferences, it is likely that the symbol of the Christmas tree will play a role in your family celebrations.

Making a Cloth Christmas Tree

Some people like to make their own Christmas trees from cloth. Making a cloth tree is not as difficult as it might sound to the novice, but careful planning is necessary.

Most cloth trees are not full size but are smaller replicas. Often they fulfill the need for a Christmas tree in places where people lack the space for a larger tree. They can be most practical for small apartments or mobile homes.

Your cloth Christmas tree will probably stand anywhere from 1 to 3 feet high. In order for the tree to have its form, two things are crucial:

❀ A tree stand to support the tree.
❀ A branch-skeletal structure to support the boughs.

The tree stand is located at the base of the tree. It can be made of anything from wood to metal to plastic. If you use plastic or lightweight metal, add weights to help keep the tree from tipping over. Wood and heavy metal are usually better choices for a stand.

The branch skeletal structure usually consists of a central wooden pole and wire branches. Some people prefer to make the whole tree out of wire, but wood is stiffer and stands up better to wear. Some like to paint or stain the central pole to help create the illusion of a real tree.

The cloth boughs are often made from rags. Usually people dye the boughs green, but some people prefer the "quilt-like" effect of the plain rags. That choice is up to your personal preference, or you might want to have your whole family vote on the matter. (You can always make more than one tree if family members can't decide on their color preferences.)

Wrap cloth tightly over wire. Be careful to not cut your fingers. Usually it works best to wrap the wire boughs *before* hanging them on your tree. There is less chance of getting scratched by wires that way, and it will be easier to hang the boughs where you want them. If you wire the tree before wrapping the boughs, you have to move the wires around so that you can get in and out to wrap each bough properly.

Small children should *not* wrap bare wire. Older children may do so under adult supervision. Keep a first-aid kit and bandages on hand.

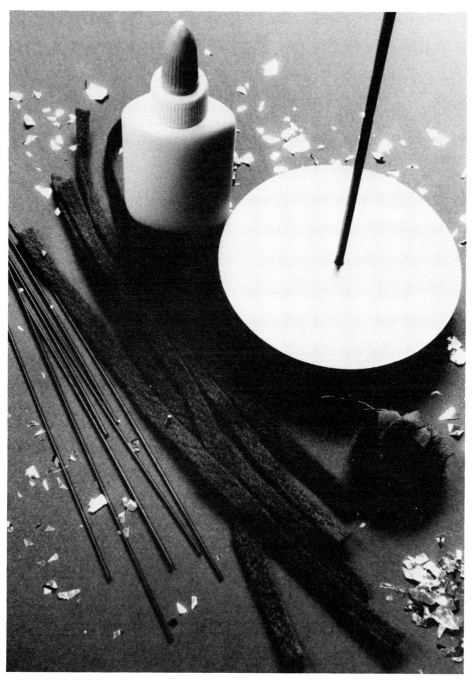

Materials for making a cloth Christmas tree.

Use only clean (rust-free) wire and wrap boughs tightly around the wire. Stitch the boughs together by hand. That will prevent them from slipping off and exposing bare wire. Some people like to tie boughs on. However, prying little hands love to untie things, so it is usually wiser to sew the boughs. Again, it is best to sew them before you hang them on the tree.

Adults or older children who possess patience and skill should be the ones to hook boughs onto the tree and position branches. Small children are not usually as coordinated as older children and adults. Also, it is best if the finished tree resembles a tree. It probably won't if you let junior put the branches on. Assign tasks that are reasonable according to ages and abilities.

If the kids make an error, help them to fix it. Don't respond with anger or criticism. If you exercise patience and love, it will make for a memorable family experience. If, on the other hand, you holler at or spank erring children, you can't expect youngsters to want to ever do this (or any other family activities) again. Children need patience and positive reinforcement. Punishment or humiliation can injure fragile bodies and egos. Remember that nobody is born knowing how to do anything. Everything is learned. So take the time to make learning fun!

Built-in Scents

The delightful thing about making a cloth Christmas tree is that you have a scent built into the tree. An easy way is to use an aromatic wood for the center and base. Cedar has a nice fragrance. There are two ways you can scent the boughs. One way is to use volatile oils, such as pine. Apply these to the fabric and let it dry before wrapping the wire branches. A second method is to sew sachet strips and use them to wrap boughs.

CLOTH CHRISTMAS TREE SACHET

5 ounces cornstarch
3 ounces talc
1 ounce powdered benzoin gum
1 drop pine oil
1 drop bergamot oil
1/4 teaspoon nutmeg
1/2 teaspoon cinnamon

CHRISTMAS DECORATIONS

One of the true joys of Christmas is the hanging of decorations on the Christmas tree. In many households this is a family event, a tradition in which all members of the family, young and old, partake. Think how even more delightful it will be when you hang your homemade decorations!

When you make the decorations, allow small children to help pick out the designs you use. Santa Claus and his reindeer are perennial favorites with most kids. Older children might be able to help you make the pot-pourri and sachet decorations. Don't forget that young children can do simple tasks. Include them whenever possible

What you choose to make to hang on your tree will depend upon your family traditions and preferences. Commercial sewing patterns are available for many cloth figurines and articles. Santa, his elves, the reindeer, candy canes, bells, stars, angels, and so many more designs are possible. If you are artistic you can draw your own sewing patterns. For sources of commercial sewing patterns, see the back of this book. You will find companies listed that sell both patterns and also ready-to-use kits that include all the materials.

The scents you choose will depend upon your chosen designs. For example, religious themes are rarely scented with peppermint or cinnamon. Frankincense and myrrh are traditionally used for religious themes.

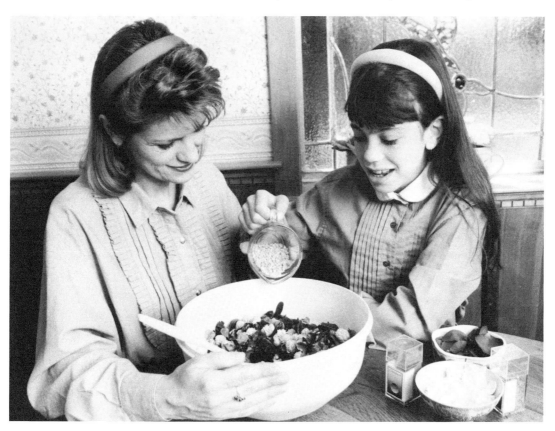

Adults should guide young helpers.

RECIPES

SANTA POTPOURRI

4 ounces peppermint leaves
2 ounces rose petals
1 ounce powdered benzoin gum
1 teaspoon vanilla
$1/2$ teaspoon cinnamon

SANTA'S REINDEER POTPOURRI

2 ounces sunbul root (smells like musk)
1 ounce heather blossoms
1 ounce powdered orris root
1 teaspoon cinnamon
$1/2$ teaspoon nutmeg
1 teaspoon vanilla

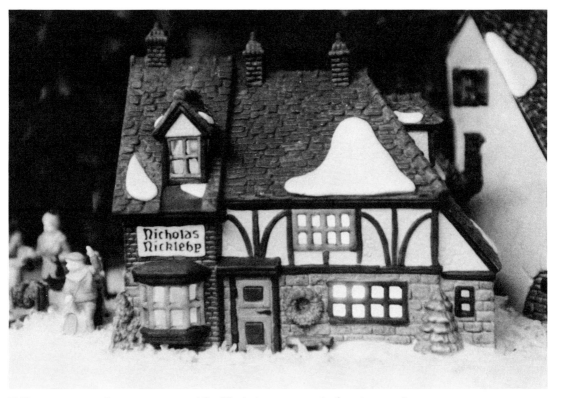

Fill commercial containers with Christmas-scented potpourris.

SANTA'S ELVES POTPOURRI

4 ounces peppermint leaves
2 ounces rose petals
1 ounce powdered benzoin gum
1 teaspoon cinnamon
1/2 teaspoon nutmeg
1 teaspoon vanilla
1 ounce lavender flowers

CANDY CANE SACHET

4 ounces cornstarch
2 ounces talc
1 ounce powdered benzoin gum
1/2 teaspoon cloves
1 teaspoon cinnamon
1/2 teaspoon nutmeg
1 drop peppermint oil
1 drop bergamot oil
1 teaspoon vanilla

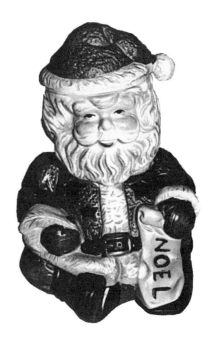

Christmas Bells

To make cloth bells ring, you must sew on tiny bells. These bells come in colors of gold, silver, red, blue, and green and can usually be found in the Christmas department of any dime store. You can also purchase them year round from specialty craft supply stores. They are economical and are usually sold in bunches on a cardboard backing in two sizes. Use the smaller size for your hanging ornaments.

BELL POTPOURRI

4 ounces rose petals
2 ounces rosemary
1 ounce deer's tongue herb
1 ounce powdered orris root
1 teaspoon nutmeg
1 teaspoon vanilla

Christmas Star

Christmas stars can be made to hang onto the tree like bells and other ornaments, or you can make a special star to hang at the top. Some people like to use elaborate embroidery, glitter, or rhinestones to decorate the top star.

STAR POTPOURRI

2 ounces geranium leaves (Rober's Lemon Rose)
2 ounces geranium leaves (Countess of Scarborough,
     strawberry-scent)
1 teaspoon vanilla
1 ounce powdered orris root
1 ounce rosemary

SANTA'S SLEIGH POTPOURRI

2 ounces rose petals
2 ounces gardenia blossoms
2 ounces peppermint leaves
1 ounce lavender
1 ounce spearmint leaves
1 teaspoon nutmeg
$1/2$ teaspoon cinnamon
1 teaspoon vanilla

After-Christmas Storage

After Christmas, always store hanging potpourri ornaments in tightly-sealed containers in a cool, dry location. Proper storage will help to prolong the aromatic qualities of your potpourri so you can enjoy them for many Christmases to come.

SCENTED PHOTO HOLDERS

It is the custom in some families to hang pictures of all of the family members on the Christmas tree. Often cloth or wooden photo holders are made specifically for this purpose. You can make your own scented variety of wood or cloth.

Wooden photo holders are easiest to make. Select an aromatic wood, such as cedar or sandalwood, saw it to size, drill a hole in the top for putting the string or yarn, and glue the picture onto the wood. Rough edges should be sanded to prevent slivers (and for aesthetic reasons). Do not varnish the wood; you might destroy the natural aroma of the wood. As time goes by, you might want to add essential oils, if the wood needs it, to create a stronger bouquet.

Cloth photo holders are really sachet pillows designed to cushion the picture and to frame it. Be sure to measure the picture so that it will fit in the desired area. Elastic straps can help secure the photo in place at the edges. Use lace or brightly-colored yarns to frame the photo. Green and red are very popular colors at Christmastime, but feel free to use your favorites.

Have family members participate in choosing the yarns and scents they like best for their own picture. Older children might be able to actually help in sewing the sachets. Younger children, although probably not as much help as they'd like to be, should be praised lavishly for their efforts.

The more you make this and other family projects to be something special, the more all will enjoy it, including yourself. So be patient and enjoy the time you have with your loved ones. Let this be a special time for all of the family, and don't forget to involve each member in a very special way.

CHRISTMAS STOCKINGS

Hanging Christmas stockings by the fireplace is still a custom in many parts of the world. It isn't as common as it once was—in part because many of today's homes no longer have fireplaces. Nevertheless, millions of people the world over still hang up Christmas stockings.

You can add sachet pillows in the form of patches to your Christmas stockings—a delightful way to add to the festive mood. Small, slender sachet pillows are made from a tightly woven fabric. They can then be sewn onto the stockings, by hand or by machine, to look as if they were patches. They are usually sewn onto the heel or toe areas to complete the effect. These sachet patches should contain only a small amount of sachet powder so they don't appear too lumpy.

FESTIVE CHRISTMAS STOCKING SACHET

4 ounces cornstarch
2 ounces talc
1 ounce powdered benzoin gum
1 teaspoon nutmeg
1/2 teaspoon cloves
1 1/2 teaspoons cinnamon
1 teaspoon vanilla
1 drop peppermint oil

Real vanilla is preferable to imitation. If using an imitation, double the amount the recipe calls for.

WILDFLOWER CHRISTMAS STOCKING SACHET

4 ounces potato starch
2 ounces talc
1 ounce powdered orris root
1 teaspoon ground rosemary
1 teaspoon cinnamon
1 drop violet oil
1 drop lemon oil

WALK-IN-THE-BLACK-FOREST SACHET

4 ounces potato starch
2 ounces talc
1 ounce powdered benzoin gum
1 teaspoon ground rue
1 teaspoon ground balsam fir needles
1 drop pine oil
1 drop lemon oil
1 teaspoon vanilla

GINGERBREAD HOUSE

Another fun family project is to make a gingerbread house potpourri. You can make a small one out of cloth to use as a tree ornament, or you can fill a larger one with Christmas fragrance. Either way, the kids will love it, and it will be a conversation piece at your holiday gatherings. You may use a commercial sewing pattern or design your own. Let the kids help with those extra decorating touches.

GINGERBREAD HOUSE POTPOURRI

2 ounces rosebuds and petals
1 ounce lavender flowers
1 ounce powdered orris root
1 tablespoon brown sugar
1 tablespoon ginger
1 teaspoon vanilla
1 drop bergamot oil

NATIVITY SCENES

Nativity scenes are a tradition in many households. If they are in yours, you may want to consider adding fragrance to your Nativity scene. One way is to make Nativity pieces out of potpourri. You can find patterns to create your models or, if you are artistic, you can design your own.

A second and easier method is simply to add fragrance to an existing set by placing sachets and potpourri in strategic locations within the scene. Usually the sachet and potpourri are disguised so that they blend in with the scene—for example, a sachet packet can be hidden under the straw in the manger or woven into the cloaks worn by the wise men.

ANIMAL POTPOURRI

2 ounces sunbal root
1 ounce sweet woodruff
1 ounce lavender flowers
1 ounce benzoin gum
1/4 teaspoon cinnamon

THREE KINGS SACHET

4 ounces cornstarch
2 ounces talc
1 teaspoon ground myrrh
2 teaspoons ground frankincense
1 teaspoon vanilla
1/2 ounce powdered sandalwood (fixative)

MANGER POTPOURRI

1 ounce sweet woodruff
1 ounce German rue
1 ounce heather blossoms
2 ounces rose petals
1 ounce powdered orris root
1 drop bergamot oil

RESTORING OLD POTPOURRI

As the years go by, many of your potpourris will lose some of their aromatic potency. Although potpourri is easily replaced, you might want to keep the originals for sentimental reasons. Fortunately, potpourri fragrance can be restored.

To refreshen an old potpourri, add a drop of bergamot oil to it. The oil can seep into the mix even through a cloth covering. It will help to re-awaken spices and floral scents long lost to time.

Time might diminish aromas during this restoration process; so while it won't work forever, it will work for a surprising number of years. Be careful, though—the scent of bergamot can become predominant if used continuously or with a heavy hand. The best way to preserve the aromatic qualities of your potpourris and sachets is to store them in airtight containers when not in use.

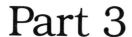

Part 3

Heated Fragrances

Chapter 8

Hot Potpourri

HOT POTPOURRI is becoming very popular. Heating potpourri helps effuse the fragrance throughout a room much faster than when potpourri is not heated. For this reason it is in demand, especially by people who are in a hurry to get results.

Potpourri that is heated will not have as long of a shelf life as regular potpourris, primarily for two reasons:

✿ Heating evaporates volatile essential oils.
✿ Heat gradually causes the physical breakdown of the individual potpourri ingredients.

Regardless, an affluent society that demands instant aromas has discovered the obvious advantages of hot potpourri.

SELECTING POTPOURRI HEATERS

Potpourri heaters come in a wide selection of shapes and sizes and are made from many materials, such as ceramic, glass, or metal. They also come with a wide range of price tags. You can purchase one for a few dollars or several hundred, depending upon your budget.

Potpourri heaters consist of three basic parts:

✿ The container that holds the potpourri.
✿ The base that holds the potpourri container.
✿ A heating unit, usually a candle that goes into the base under the container.

While all heaters require these three basic parts, the number of designs for potpourri heaters are vast and impressive. You might want to select a model that fits the decor of the room in which you plan to use it.

Or, if gift-giving is what you have in mind, try to match your gift with the personality of the recipient. For example, if someone favors Victorian artifacts, they might not appreciate a "contemporary" model. Common sense is the best guide to selecting gifts. If in doubt, do your homework. Remember: It is a good idea never to pick out for a gift something that you wouldn't like yourself.

Ceramic Heaters. Of the wide assortment of potpourri heaters on the market, ceramic heaters are the most popular. Ceramic is an excellent material for heating potpourri, and can be molded into many forms. The design possibilities are almost unlimited.

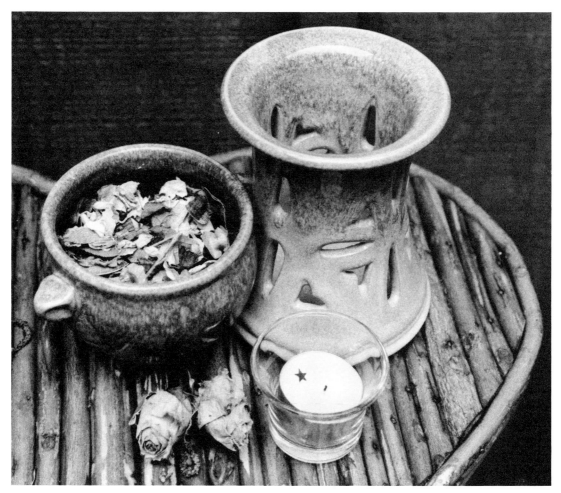

The three basic parts of a potpourri heater.

Ceramic can break, however, so it should not be displayed where small children or pets can get to it.

Glass Heaters. Slightly more fragile than ceramic, glass potpourri heaters are also very attractive. Those made from glass crystal are especially appealing. Glass offers the advantage of making the potpourri visible, so you can see its many-colored herbs, flowers, and spices.

Cheaper glass potpourri heaters are also available. Ones that employ colored glass are especially popular. It is best not to place potpourri heaters made from glass crystal and those made from common glass in the same room. Crystal makes plain glass look cheap in comparison.

Wood Heaters. Many fine potpourri heaters employ fine hardwoods, such as cherry, oak, or mahagony. Softwoods can also be used. However, wood can never be used for the pot that is to be heated because—obviously—wood is flammable.

Wood potpourri heaters can be made durable than either glass or ceramic, but they can also be slightly more expensive.

Metal Heaters. Some people love the look and feel of fine brass. Brass potpourri heaters are a good buy. They are attractive, durable, and won't break like glass or ceramic can.

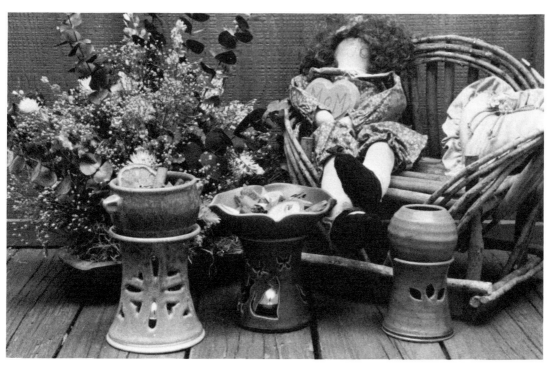

Many varieties of potpourri heaters are available.

Brass is the most popular metal; however, copper, pewter, and bronze models are also available. Most of these metals can be silver-plated or gold-plated for a rich look, or they can be left to develop a natural patina. If you like your metals to shine, you can polish them regularly with metal polish.

HOT POTPOURRI RECIPES

The only drawback to heating potpourri is that it tends to shorten the shelf life of the potpourri. On the other hand, you don't need as much potpourri when using it hot. The aromatic effects of a couple of tablespoons will equal that of a larger batch unheated.

HOT VICTORIAN PARLOR POTPOURRI

2 ounces rosebuds
2 ounces geranium leaves (Countess of Scarborough)
1 ounce granular frankincense (fixative)
1 vanilla bean
1 ounce rosemary
1 ounce rue

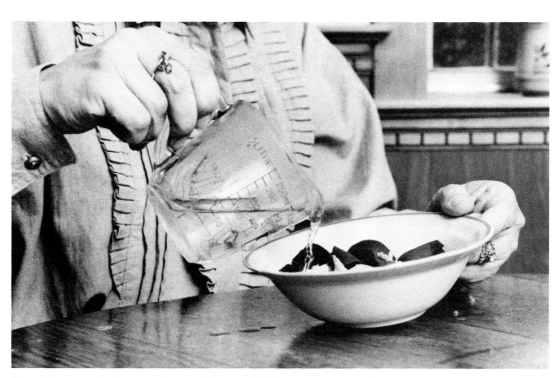

A quick way to draw out scent is to add hot water to a dry mix.

RED HOT ROSE POTPOURRI

4 ounces red rosebuds and petals
1 stick cinnamon
2 ounces rosemary
1 ounce granular benzoin gum
1 vanilla bean

HOT LAVENDER POTPOURRI

2 ounces lavender flowers
1 ounce rose petals
1 stick cinnamon
2 ounces damiana leaves
1 ounce granular myrrh gum (fixative)

HOT AMBER POTPOURRI

2 ounces granular amber resin
1 ounce granular frankincense
2 ounces rose petals (yellow roses)
2 ounces deer's tongue herb
1 vanilla bean

HOT TAJ MAHAL POTPOURRI

2 ounces sandalwood chips
2 ounces patchouli leaves
1 ounce granular frankincense (fixative)
1 stick cinnamon
1 tonka bean

HOT PIERRE POTPOURRI

4 ounces jasmine flowers
2 ounces violets
1 ounce rue
1 ounce cut orris root
1 vanilla bean

HOT GEISHA POTPOURRI

2 ounces peony blossoms
2 ounces camellia flowers
2 ounces chrysanthemum blossoms
1 ounce oleander flowers
1 ounce granular benzoin gum

HOT ΘTTO POTPOURRI

2 ounces sweet woodruff

2 ounces rue

1 ounce balsam fir needles

1 ounce cedar chips

1 ounce cut orris root

1 teaspoon nutmeg

HOT ITALIAN POTPOURRI

2 ounces majoram

1 ounce oregano

1 ounce sweet basil

1 ounce granular myrrh (fixative)

1 cinnamon stick

HOT SHANGHAI POTPOURRI

2 ounces ylang ylang

2 ounces cut gingseng root

2 ounces ma hung

1 ounce granular benzoin gum

1 tablespoon orange peel

HOT IRISH POTPOURRI

1 ounce shamrock leaves

1 ounce rosebuds

1 ounce heather

1 ounce granular amber resin (fixative)

1 drop oil of bergamot

HOT SPANISH POTPOURRI

2 ounces dried tomato pieces

1 ounce dried pimento pepper

2 ounces dried green olives

1 clove garlic

1 ounce granular benzoin gum

HOT PERSIAN POTPOURRI

2 ounces rosebuds

1 ounce poppy seeds

1 ounce damiana leaves

1 ounce gum arabic (fixative)

1 drop lilac oil

HOT ARABIAN NIGHTS POTPOURRI

2 ounces rosebuds and petals
2 ounces cedar shavings
1 ounce sandalwood shavings (fixative)
1 ounce coffee blossoms
1 stick cinnamon

HOT MEDITERRANEAN POTPOURRI

2 ounces citron
1 ounce lemon peel
2 ounces calendula flowers
1 ounce saffron blossoms
2 ounces lily-of-the-valley flowers
1 drop almond oil

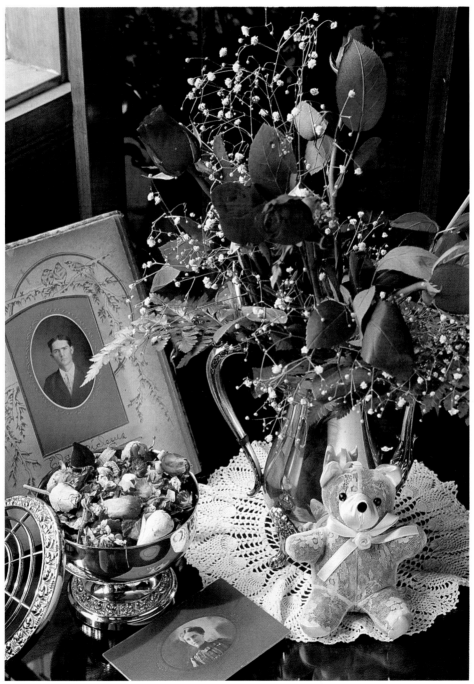

Roses of any color can be used effectively in potpourri. These red beauties can be enjoyed long after the blooms fade.

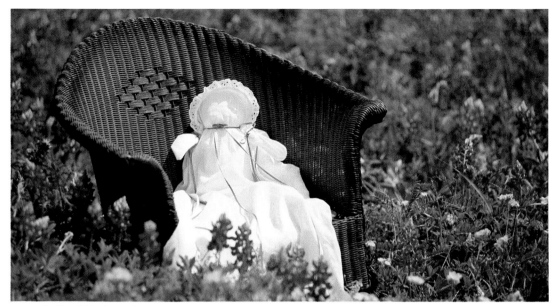

Rag dolls filled with potpourri make delightful gifts for children.

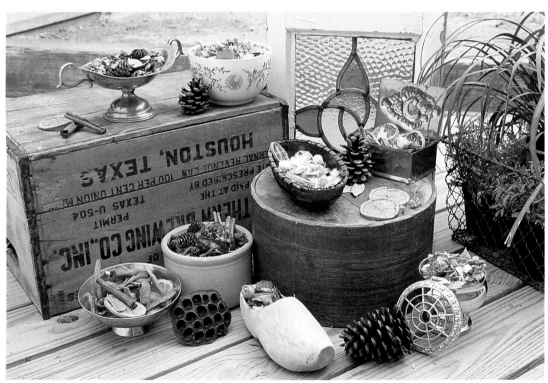

Containers for your potpourris are limited only by your imagination.

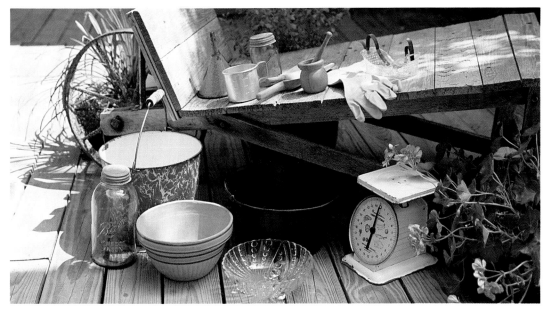

Some of the tools needed to create the wonderful homemade scents in this book.

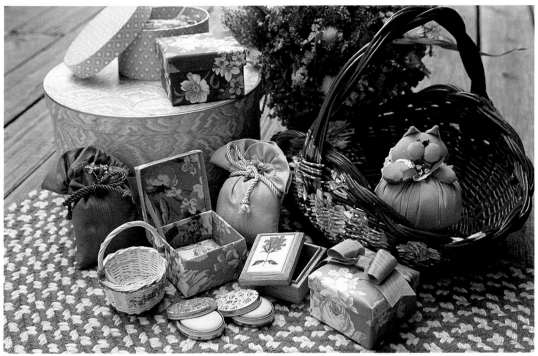

Beautiful packaging is the finishing touch for your efforts.

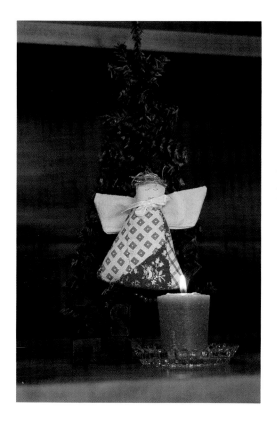

A tiny angel filled with sachet powder or potpourri adds a scented touch to your Christmas tree.

Sachet pillows secured to a rope of brightly colored yarn make an attractive, aromatic display.

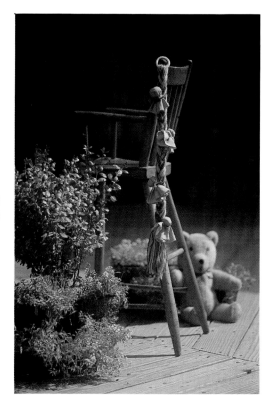

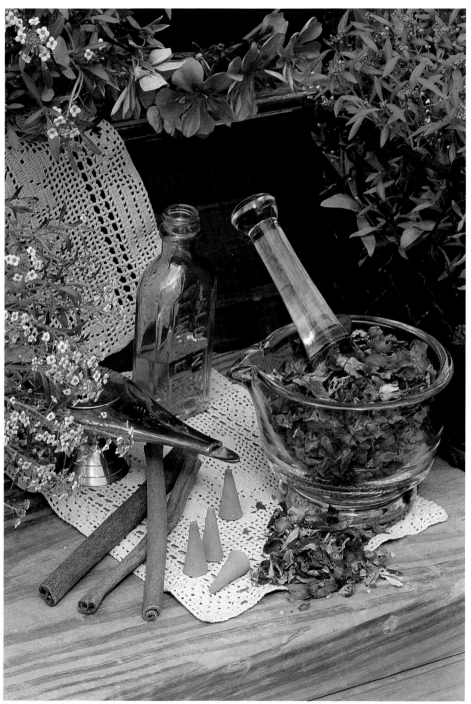

To make incense, grind all ingredients (except oils) to a fine powder.

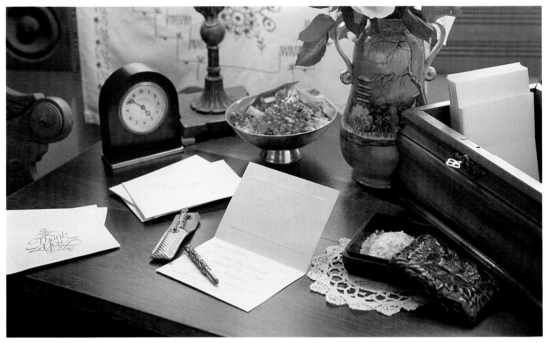

Letters and notes scented with sachet powders can be your "hallmark" to a friend or sweetheart.

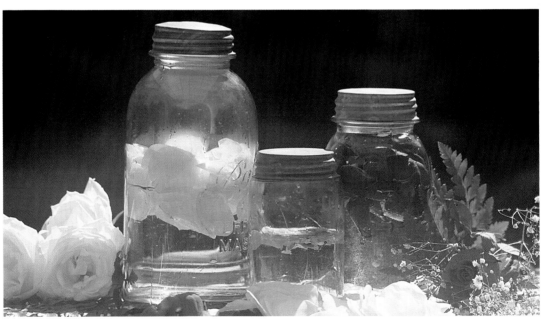

You can make cologne from fresh flowers in one sunny afternoon.

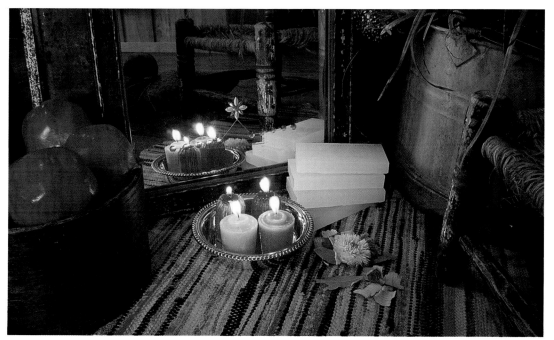

The soft glow and fragrance of candles have been enjoyed for centuries.

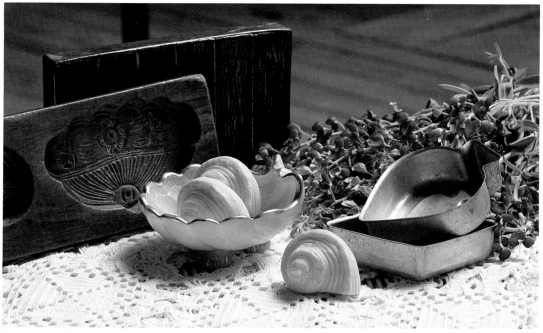

Soap can be molded into an unlimited variety of shapes and sizes.

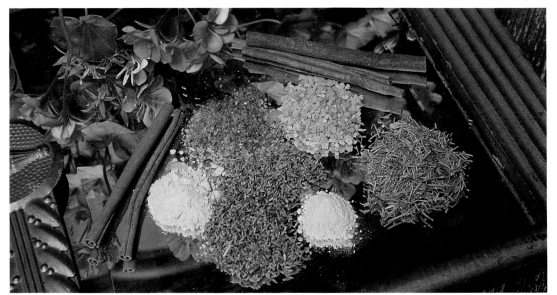

Cinnamon sticks, orris root, benzoin gum, rosemary, lavender, myrrh gum, and frankincense gum are a few ingredients for recipes in this book.

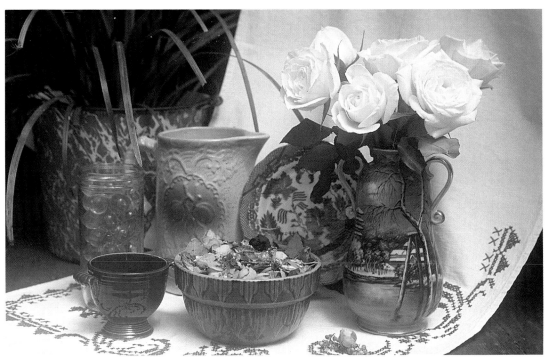

Rose petals make wonderful potpourri, cologne, sachet, and incense for your home.

Chapter 9

Scented Candles

PEOPLE HAVE LIT CANDLES for centuries as part of spiritual ritual or to mask offensive odors. Many ancients added fragrant ingredients to their candles which made the lighting of them more pleasant. During the Black Plague, small amounts of sulfur were often added to candles to help cleanse the air of the poisons of the plague.

Making candles is much easier these days than in times past. So many aids to candle making are available commercially. Nowadays paraffin wax is used extensively; it is cheaper to buy than tallow and readily available. Also, because it is already a wax, paraffin need only be reheated and poured into a mold to take the desired shape.

WAXES

Many types of waxes can be useful in making candles. Paraffin and beeswax are the most popular types.

Paraffin. Paraffin wax doesn't come from animal sources, which might please some people. It is a by-product of the petroleum industry. (If that thought disturbs you, other options are available.)

Paraffin comes in plain white blocks. It is the cheapest wax to buy. However, it melts quickly, so you'll want to coat your candles with a thin layer of beeswax if you want longer burning candles.

Beeswax. The best candles are made from beeswax or from a combination of waxes that utilizes beeswax as a pivotal element. Beeswax melts slowly. It gives a nice, steady flame. However, beeswax is more expensive, so it is usually used as a coating, or in combination with cheaper waxes.

Tropical Waxes. *Carnuba* and *palm* waxes can also be used to make candles, but they produce very hard candles unless used in combination with other, softer waxes. Coating paraffin candles with a layer of carnuba wax will give them a longer burn life.

FATS

Candles can also be made from fats. Historically, they've been made from tallow and sometimes lard, but they can also be made from hydrogenated vegetable shortening. One of the problems with candles made of fat is that they tend to get soft at room temperature and really soften when they get warm. Hot candles will melt rapidly. Candles made purely from fats may get too soft if set out in a warm room.

One way to solve this problem is by keeping candles in the refrigerator when you're not using them. Tallow is naturally firmer than lard or hydrogenated vegetable shortening, but it, too, will soften.

A more practical solution is to coat candles with a layer of carnuba wax or beeswax to give them a tougher outer shell and to allow the candle

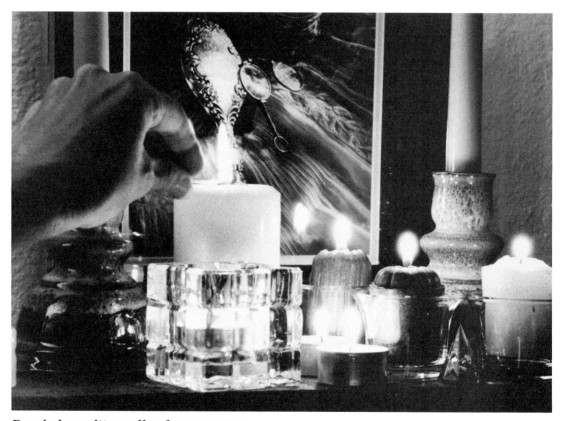

People have lit candles for centuries.

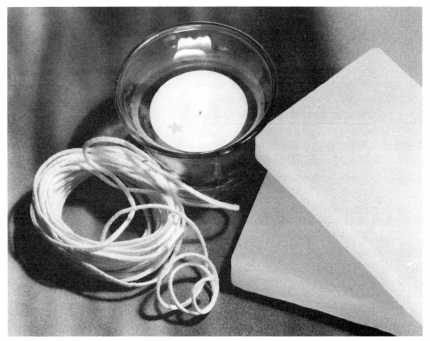

Making candles is easier these days than in times past.

to keep its shape. Your candle will then burn slower and won't get mushy or start to wilt everytime it gets warm in the house.

In most cases, mixing a portion of wax right into the candles will also improve the qualities of the candle.

Advantages of Using Fats

The primary advantage to using fats is that they are readily available, and shortening is reasonably inexpensive. A can of shortening can yield a lot of candles. However *never* reuse candle fat in foods.

Another advantage of using vegetable fat is that it is very easy to work with—easier than wax because it is already soft. However, better candles are made when wax is added to the mix, or used to coat the outside of the candle.

COLORS

Some people favor candles with just the natural color of their ingredients, but usually coloring is added to provide variety and appeal. Candles made without adding a colorant will take on the color of the principal ingredients: Candles made from paraffin will be white; those made from beeswax, a warm ivory; and those from tallow, a pale yellow. You might want to leave some of your candles natural to contrast to the colored ones, but you'll probably want to color some, especially if you are making candles for market.

Chemical Colorants

One of the two primary ways to add color to your candles is to use chemical dyes. These dyes are mostly coal tar derivatives. Food-grade dyes available at any supermarket do the job nicely.

Chemical colorants produce bright, sharp colors, very uniform in tint from batch to batch. Usually only a few drops will suffice to create the color you desire. Colors can also be mixed to create new hues and tints. Chemical colorants are quite reasonably priced.

Chemical colorants do have some drawbacks. One is that colors are so bright: If you favor pastel shades, you really have to be careful not to use too much of a colorant. Because of their brightness, clarity of color, and the uniformity of the batches, chemical colorants create an artificial look, as few things in nature are quite that uniform. A second, perhaps more important, drawback is that some people vehemently object to products colored with artificial colorants. If you are making candles for market, this is a reality you might have to confront. The coloring agents that you use to color your candles and other scented products might make the difference in securing a sale.

Herbal Colorants

The other way to add color to candles is with herbal colorants. Herbal colorants were used long before the invention of modern chemical dyes.

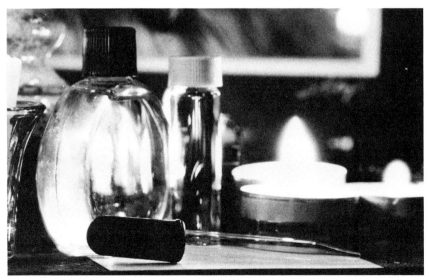

Use only a drop or two of essential oils for a rich perfume.

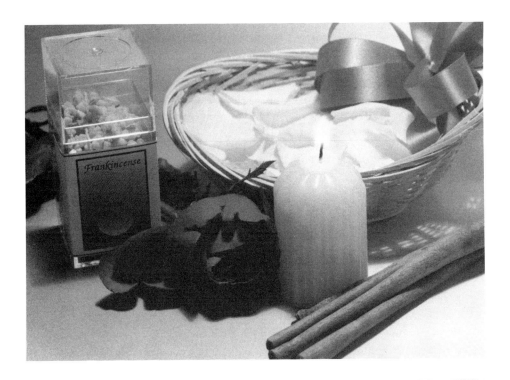

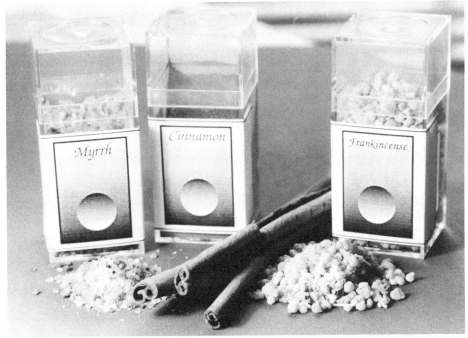

Many ingredients can be used to scent your candles.

They produce candles just like our ancestors did. One of the advantages of herbal colorants is they look more natural, more in tune with the hues of nature. Another advantage is that herbally colored products are growing in popularity and can boost sales.

Some of the disadvantages of herbal colorants are the same as the advantages. For example, herbal colorants produce more muted colors than do their chemical counterparts. Anyone who really wants sharper colors should use a chemical colorant.

Another disadvantage is cost. Herbs cost more than chemical colorants (unless you grow your own). Also, there will be less uniformity of color between batches and, to a lesser degree, within batches.

Some of the usual herbal colorants are:

RED—beets, henna, or cochineal.
BLUE—woad, or indigo.
SCARLET—madder root.
GREEN—indigo combined with safflower.
YELLOW—goldenrod, safflower.
ORANGE—annatto seed.
LAVENDER—black malva flowers
BROWN—catechu (from India), butternut, or black walnut.
BLACK—alderbark and logwood, or red hibiscus flowers.

Adding Colorants

Colors should be worked into the softened wax (and/or fats) so that the colorant is evenly dispersed within the mixture. This is very important to giving candles a uniform color. Add colorant while the mixture is in a liquid state, just before removing it from the heat. Do not continue to heat the mixture with the colorant in it, or it can adversely affect the color of the final product.

If you are planning to coat your candles with beeswax, you have the option of just adding color to the beeswax, coloring both, or coloring the base candle and leaving the beeswax coating uncolored. You can also color each with a contrasting color, such as red and yellow, blue and green, etc. You might wish to vary your practice for a variety of effects that you can achieve.

Follow each recipe for exact coloring to avoid the embarrassment of different batches being different color shades. Remember that if you are using an herbal colorant, you will still likely have a greater variety of hues than you'd get from a chemical colorant. This isn't crucial most of the time, but in sales, people tend to expect uniformity in the goods they buy. If one time they purchase a candle from you that is cherry red and the next time the same candle is brick red, your customers might find it upsetting—especially when people think they are buying candles that will match a set. If the colors are off, so is the symmetry.

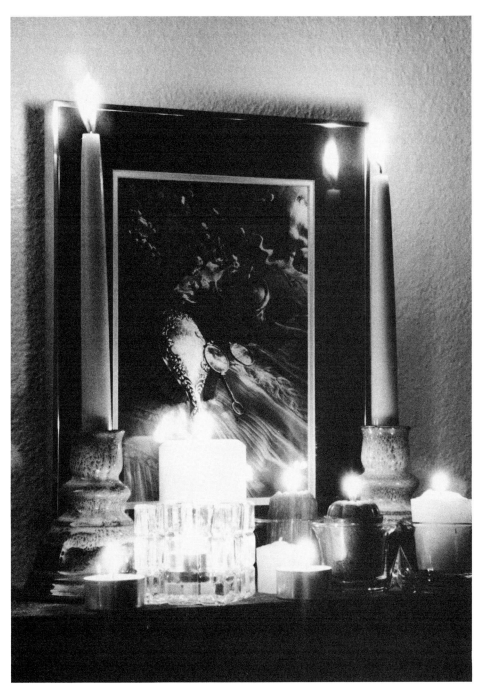

Candles can be formed into many shapes and sizes.

CANDLE RECIPES

Candle recipes differ according to the ingredients used. In all recipes it is important that fragrance is added as the *last* ingredient, after the colorant.

Use of essential oils is the preferred way to scent candles because they won't affect the color of the finished product. However, powdered herbs, gums, and even rose petals can also be added for fragrance.

When adding any fragrance, stir the mixture to thoroughly diffuse the scent throughout the entire mixture. Add fragrances last, just before the wax starts to harden. Never add floral or other essential oils to boiling wax, or you will likely lose most of the fragrance before the candle hardens.

PLAIN WHITE PARAFFIN CANDLES

1 pound paraffin wax
1/4 yard candlewick or twine
2 drops almond oil

Heat wax in kettle over a slow burner; stir to prevent scorching. Cut candlewick to desired lengths and position in the candle molds. Be careful to center the wicks to the best of your ability. This will help the candles to burn evenly. Remove hot wax from heat. Stir air into it to help cool it off. Add fragrance just before pouring into the molds. Stir thoroughly to disperse the fragrance. Pour into molds when the mixture has the consistency of gravy.

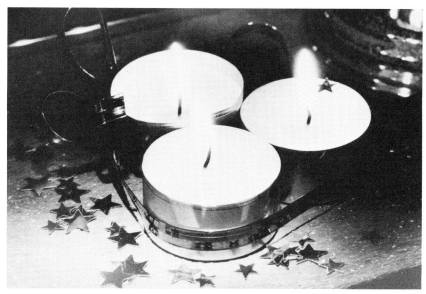

Small candles are an ideal gift.

YELLOW PARAFFIN CANDLES

1 pound paraffin wax
$1/4$ yard candlewick or twine
2 tablespoons powdered goldenrod
2 drops lemon oil

Add more colorant if a deeper shade is desired. Follow the directions for plain paraffin candles.

RED PARAFFIN CANDLES

1 pound paraffin wax
$1/4$ yard candlewick or twine
2 tablespoons beet powder
1 teaspoon vanilla
3 teaspoons cinnamon

PLAIN BEESWAX CANDLES

1 pound beeswax
$1/4$ yard candlewick or twine
2 drops almond oil

Heat wax in kettle on a slow burner. Stir to prevent scorching. Cut candlewick to desired lengths, and center them in candle molds to keep candles even. Remove hot wax from heat; stir in air to cool wax. Add fragrance, stirring to disperse it evenly. Pour into candle molds when the mixture has the consistency of gravy. Candles will be a warm ivory in color.

BLACK BEESWAX CANDLES

1 pound beeswax
$1/4$ yard candlewick or twine
2 tablespoons red hibiscus flowers (powdered)
2 drops anise oil

Beeswax-Coated Candles

Most of the candles you make will probably be with a paraffin base and beeswax coating because this is one of the cheapest ways to make a quality candle. It is much more economical than using beeswax alone, and it makes a longer lasting candle than those made from pure paraffin.

When coating paraffin with beeswax, you have several options as to what color effects you wish to create. For example, you can color the beeswax and leave the paraffin uncolored. Or you can color the paraffin and leave the beeswax uncolored (which, incidentally, mutes the brighter colors of chemical colorants). Or you can color them both the same color, contrasting colors, or hues that harmonize on the color scheme.

Another area of choice is whether to scent both waxes with the same scent, or with a harmonious scent. (You don't want conflicting scents, such as frankincense and peppermint.) You can also choose to scent only the beeswax, or only the paraffin.

RED BEESWAX OVER WHITE PARAFFIN CANDLES

1 pound paraffin wax
1/4 pound beeswax
1/4 yard candlewick
2 drops rose oil

Heat beeswax in separate kettle from the paraffin wax, *after* the paraffin wax has already been poured into molds and hardened. Remove candles from molds and dip them quickly into the beeswax so that it evenly coats the candles. Repeated dippings might be necessary.

Never dip candles into hot wax. The beeswax should be the consistency of gravy. If the wax gets too thick, reheat it and start over. Use metal tongs when handling candles. Hot wax is dangerous and can cause severe burns. Be careful to not splatter it on you and keep all distractions, including children and pets out of the room while the mixture is hot. The candle will be most fragrant if the wax closest to the burning wick is scented.

Mixed Wax Candles

You can also mix waxes to obtain candles with some of the qualities of each individual wax. Some people find this easier than coating the candles. For softer candles, you can add vegetable fats, but be sure to use the proper ratio of ingredients.

MIXED WAX CANDLE RECIPES

PEACH CANDLES

1/2 pound paraffin
1/4 pound beeswax
1/4 yard candlewick
2 tablespoons powdered annatto seed
1/2 teaspoon powdered madder root
2 drops peach oil

HYACINTH CANDLES

1/2 pound paraffin wax
1/4 pound beeswax
1/4 yard candlewick
1 tablespoon black malva flowers (powdered)
1/2 teaspoon cochineal
2 drops hyacinth oil

LAVENDER CANDLES

$1/2$ pound paraffin
$1/4$ pound beeswax
2 tablespoons black malva flowers (powdered)
2 drops lavender oil
$1/4$ yard candlewick or twine

Powdered Aromatic Additives

FRANKINCENSE AND MYRRH CANDLES

$1/2$ pound paraffin
$1/4$ pound beeswax
$1/4$ yard candlestick
1 ounce powdered myrrh
1 ounce powdered frankincense
2 tablespoons powdered saffron

Heat waxes together in kettle over a slow burner. Stir to blend waxes and prevent scorching. Cut candlewick to desired lengths, and position it in the candle molds. Center wicks so that the candles will burn evenly. Remove hot wax from stove; stir in air. Add coloring agent and stir to dispense colorant uniformly. Add powdered fragrances. Stir thoroughly. Pour mixture into molds when it has the consistency of gravy.

AMBER RESIN CANDLES

$1/2$ pound paraffin
$1/4$ pound beeswax
$1/4$ yard candlewick
2 ounces powdered amber resin
2 tablespoons annatto (powdered seed)

SANDALWOOD CANDLES

$1/2$ pound paraffin wax
$1/4$ pound beeswax
2 ounces powdered sandalwood
1 tablespoon catechu
2 teaspoons powdered safflowers

CEDAR CANDLES

$1/2$ pound paraffin
$1/4$ pound beeswax
$1/4$ yard candlewick
2 ounces powdered cedar
2 tablespoons powdered black walnut husks

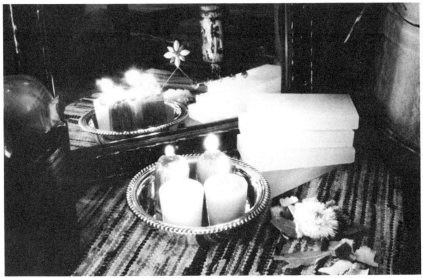

You can use spices and herbs to scent your candles.

PLAIN WHITE VEGETABLE FAT CANDLES

1 pound hydrogenated shortening (Crisco)
$1/4$ yard candlewick
2 drops almond oil

Heat shortening in kettle to soften. Cut candlewick to desired lengths, and center wicks in candle molds to keep candles burning evenly. Remove shortening from heat. Stir in fragrance, mixing thoroughly. Pour into candle molds. For best results store candles in the refrigerator or freezer. Short, fat candles hold up better than tall, thin types. Your candles will be soft and have a greasy feel to them. Avoid handling them any more than you have to, as they will soften more from your body heat. Pick them up gently with tongs and carry them in holders.

Mixed Wax and Fat Candles

Vegetable fat candles can be coated with wax to give them a longer burning life and help them keep their shape better in a warm room.

Another possible answer is to mix fats and waxes. The result is a higher quality candle than with fats alone, but these candles are usually not as good as plain wax candles. Carnuba wax can be used to produce a harder candle.

WAX AND FAT CANDLE

$1/2$ pound shortening
$1/4$ pound carnuba wax
$1/4$ yard candlewick
2 drops almond oil

Chapter 10

Incense

THE BURNING OF INCENSE has been a part of religious ceremonies since ancient times. It is still practiced in the Orient, while in the Western world the use of incense is primarily restricted to ceremonies within the Roman Catholic and Eastern Orthodox churches, and among those Westerners who practice Eastern religions (Buddhists, Hindus, Jains, etc.).

The burning of incense was never officially incorporated into the Anglican church, nor into most Protestant sects, although services in individual churches do vary.

The Crusaders brought incense back from the Middle East. During much of the Middle Ages, (and even some today) burning incense was associated with magic, including black magic or witchcraft. Today, burning incense can be enjoyed in a secular setting.

HOW INCENSE IS MADE

Incense is made from a number of gums, resins, woods, and spices. Traditional recipes include such gums as frankincense, myrrh, and camphor; such woods as sandalwood, cedar, cinnamon, and balsam; and such spices as cloves and nutmeg. Flowers and herbs have also been used in incense, especially saffron and roses, and sweet woodruff and dragon's blood. Almost any fragrant herb, flower, gum, wood, or resin can be used to make incense.

Fixative Agents

All incense recipes require a fixative agent. What these fixative agents do is to fix an incense so that the volatile oils that provide most of the aromatic qualities remain within the incense. If you didn't use a fixative agent, your incense would lose its scent before it was even lit. Fortunately many gums, resins, and some woods act as fixative agents. These include: benzoin gum, orris root, sandalwood, frankincense, myrrh gum, gum arabic, and others.

Benzoin gum and *orris root* are most commonly selected as fixative agents, the others are highly aromatic and can conflict with your chosen fragrance. (Naturally, if you want sandalwood incense, you can simply use sandalwood, and so on.) Benzoin gum has a slight woodsy odor, while orris root resembles the fragrance of voilets and is preferred for floral incenses.

Making a Powder

To make incense, grind all ingredients (except for liquids) to a fine powder. There are two primary reasons for this:

- ❀ There is a better dispersion of materials in powder form, integrating the aromatic qualities.
- ❀ The incense will be molded, and it is easier to mold a powder than granular or chunky ingredients, which don't hold together as well as powder does.

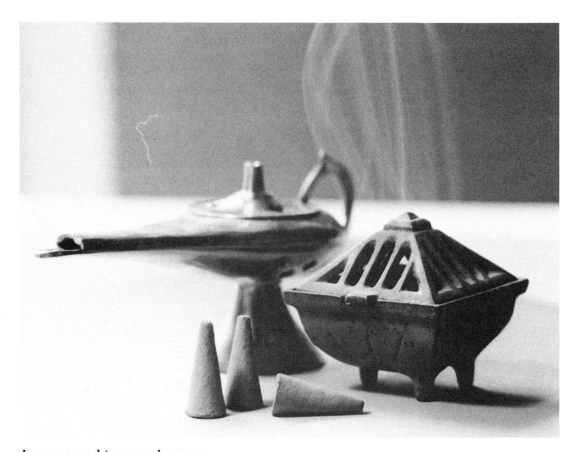

Incense and incense burners.

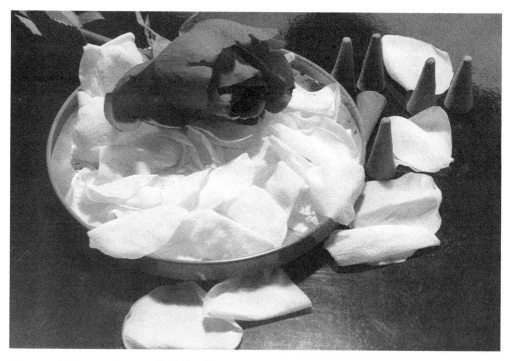

Rose petals can be made into incense.

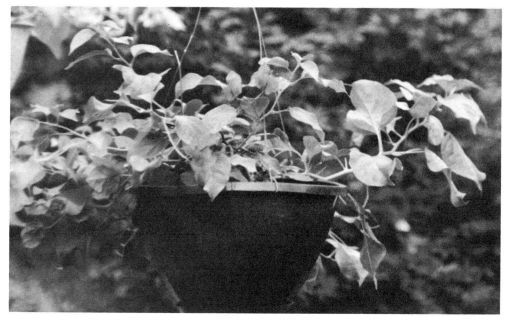

You can grow your own plants for making incense.

Use a mortar and pestle to grind all dry ingredients to as fine a powder as possible. Grind each ingredient separately, then dump them all into a larger glass or steel bowl. Proceed accordingly with each ingredient.

Naturally, the fresher your ingredients, the better quality your incense will be. If possible, use fresh spices and grind them just before using them so they have a more potent aroma than powdered spices that have been ground for some time.

Once you have all the dry ingredients in your recipe, mix them thoroughly. Stir so that the various ingredients are as evenly blended as possible, then add your fixative agent, which should also be in a powdered form. Mix it in well.

Adding Liquids

Once your dry incense powder is ready, you will add the liquid ingredients. Use an eyedropper set aside for this purpose. (Once an eyedropper has been used for scenting products, *never* use it for the eyes.) The eyedropper is necessary to carefully measure the amount of liquids added. If you add too much liquid, you will ruin your recipe. Only a small amount of liquid vegetable oil should be added to help form the paste. Olive oil is traditional, but any liquid oil will do. (Avoid motor oils; they could start a fire).

Add just enough liquid to form a paste, usually only a few drops. Keep working it with your spoon so that all of the powder is now a thick paste.

Your incense is now ready for shaping. You can shape your incense in a number of ways: by hand, with a roller pin or a cookie cutter, or using special molds purchased for the purpose. Incense is usually shaped in the form of a small cone or rod. It is burned from one end to the other.

Very tiny cones supply a great deal of fragrance, so avoid making large cakes of incense. You want to burn incense to release a small amount of aromatic smoke to create atmosphere, not to gag everyone out of the building!

You can shape incense cones by hand, but it is less time-consuming to use a mold; plus, you'll get more uniform results. Remember, people expect the products they purchase to be uniform in size.

Other Ingredients

Sugar. Sugar is not a necessary ingredient, but some people like to use it to sweeten their incense. This is especially helpful with heavy odors such as myrrh.

Sometimes powdered sugar is used for shaping the paste into rods or cones. It helps to keep the paste from sticking to your fingers.

Oils. While you can use any liquid vegetable oil, avoid using oils that are highly scented, such as peanut oil or cod liver oil. These highly scented oils will likely impart odors of their own into your incense, ruining the aromatic quality of your product in almost every case.

Olive and linseed oils work nicely and are usually available at the supermarket. Because you will only need a miniscule amount of oil in your incense recipes, you might simply borrow the oil from a neighbor if you are out of it yourself.

Flour. Some people use plain white flour as a dustcovering for incense. It helps keep the paste from sticking to their fingers when they are trying to shape the cones or rods—Anyone who bakes can tell you that!

DRYING INCENSE

Your incense must be dried and hardened before it is ready for use. It can be dried in the sun, at low heat in your oven, or in a vegetable dehydrator if you have one. Your incense is ready when it can hold its form without the mold and is completely dry with no traces of oil. Be careful to not squeeze your incense even when it is dry or you might crush it. After all, it isn't made from cement.

If you dry incense in a conventional oven, use the lowest setting and check it after five to ten minutes. You want to dry your cones, not bake them. The longer they are in the oven, the more fragrance is being lost.

You can dry incense in the sun or on a sunny windowsill. It might take longer, but it is the traditional way to dry incense. Some people believe that solar-dried incense maintains a higher aromatic potency than incense that is oven-dried.

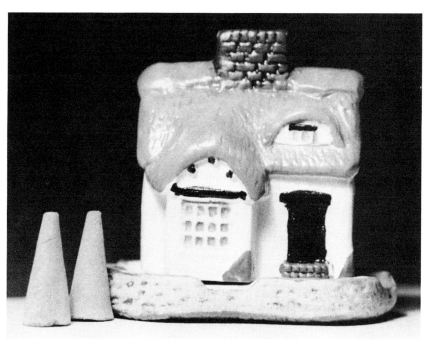

Cones of incense work well in ceramic burners.

STORING INCENSE

An important part of keeping incense, as with all scented products, is proper storage. Store in a cool, dry location, preferably in a secure area where little children or pets will not have access to it. A small child trying to light an incense cone can start a fire, and very tiny children like to try to eat everything.

Incense that is stored in damp areas will absorb the moisture and rapidly disintegrate over time.

Some people like to wrap each incense cone to help keep them at their potent best. You can do this if you wish, but the fixative agent in your incense should keep your incense fragrant. Wrap up all the cones of each type of incense together. Don't mix and match cones—they can interfere with the aromatic integrity of the others.

Store incense away from all foods because food can capture some of the incense odors.

RECIPES

AMBER INCENSE

1 ounce powdered amber resin
$1/4$ teaspoon powdered sugar
2 drops flaxseed oil

GOLDEN AMBER INCENSE

1 ounce powdered amber resin
$1/4$ teaspoon powdered sugar
$1/2$ teaspoon nutmeg
$1/4$ teaspoon sandalwood powder
1 drop linseed oil
1 drop bergamot oil

SANDALWOOD INCENSE

1 ounce sandalwood powder
$1/4$ teaspoon cinnamon
$1/4$ teaspoon powdered sugar
2 drops olive oil

CINNAMON INCENSE

2 sticks cinnamon (ground to a powder)
2 tablespoons powdered benzoin gum
$1/4$ teaspoon sugar (powdered)
1 drop linseed oil
1 drop vanilla

FRANKINCENSE

1 ounce frankincense powder
$1/4$ teaspoon cinnamon
$1/4$ teaspoon sugar (powdered)
2 drops olive oil

MYRRH INCENSE

1 ounce myrrh powder
$1/2$ teaspoon powdered sugar
2 drops olive oil

ROSE INCENSE

1 ounce powdered orris root
$1/4$ teaspoon powdered sugar
$1/4$ teaspoon cinnamon
1 drop rose oil
1 drop flaxseed oil

LAVENDER INCENSE

1 ounce powdered orris root
$1/4$ teaspoon sugar
1 drop lavender oil
1 drop flaxseed oil

SAFFRON INCENSE

1 ounce powdered saffron
$1/2$ ounce powdered orris root
2 drops olive oil

LILY-OF-THE-VALLEY INCENSE

1 ounce powdered orris root
$1/4$ teaspoon cinnamon
1 drop olive oil
1 drop lily-of-the-valley oil

JASMINE INCENSE

1 ounce powdered benzoin gum
$1/4$ teaspoon cinnamon
1 drop jasmine oil
1 drop bergamot oil

ROYAL JASMINE INCENSE

1 ounce powdered orris root
1/2 ounce powdered frankincense
1/4 teaspoon powdered sugar
1 drop rose oil
1 drop jasmine oil

BALSAM INCENSE

1 ounce powdered balsam
1/4 teaspoon nutmeg
1 drop bergamot oil
1 drop olive oil

NUTMEG INCENSE

2 tablespoons ground nutmeg
1 ounce powdered benzoin gum
1/4 teaspoon powdered sugar
1 drop vanilla
1 drop flaxseed oil

CLOVES INCENSE

6 cloves ground to a powder
1 ounce powdered benzoin gum
1 drop vanilla
1 drop cottonseed oil

PEPPERMINT INCENSE

1 ounce powdered benzoin gum
1/4 teaspoon sugar
1/4 teaspoon cinnamon
1 drop peppermint oil
1 drop oil of bergamot

LEMON INCENSE

1 ounce powdered orris root
1/4 teaspoon powdered sugar
1 drop lemon oil
1 drop vanilla

Note: On all incense recipes, if there is not enough oil to form the paste, use the eyedropper to add drops of water—slowly, until a paste can be formed. Be wary of using too much water; all you will likely need is a few drops to help form a thick paste.

GHEE

Another incense-like substance that comes from the Orient is called *ghee*. It was used traditionally to purify air, and it is still used in parts of India and Tibet in religious ceremonies.

Ghee is clarified butter. It is usually scented with an aromatic essence to provide a delightful, smokeless alternative to regular incense.

You will need to purchase a special ghee lamp to burn ghee. Stores that sell Indian and/or Tibetan merchandise often sell these lamps, or you can order one through a specialty mail-order firm.

How to Make Butter

You can make ghee from scratch by making butter. Simply take a pint of heavy cream (whipping cream) and churn it until it becomes butter. If you don't have cows or goats (and most Americans don't these days), you can purchase whipping cream from your grocer. Whip it with your beater or blender until it forms butter, or put it in a wide-top covered mason jar and shake it until it is stiff. Be sure to use a wide-top jar or you might have trouble removing the butter from the jar.

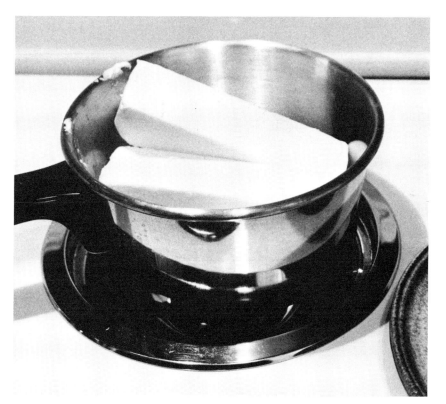

To clarify butter for ghee, melt it completely on low heat.

Most of the butter you can buy is made from sour cream, whereas the butter that you make up fresh will be sweet cream butter. You may salt it lightly if you wish, but no salt is necessary for the purpose of making ghee.

If you don't have the time to make your own butter, you can buy some at the supermarket. Be sure to use 100% butter and not a blend. Blends will contain materials that you can't use.

How to Clarify Butter

Ghee is the golden oil derived from butter after the white milk solids are removed. To remove the white milk solids (known as *clarifying*), you must heat the butter. Heat on a low burner; do not boil. The butter must melt completely.

Remove from heat, then pour the golden oil that has separated into a jar, keeping the white milk solids out.

If you set the pan down again to settle, you might be able to extract still more oil as the solids settle to the bottom of the pan. Pour off as much of the oil as possible, always keeping the white milk solids out. If any solids get into your jar, let them settle to the bottom of the jar and pour the oil into a new jar. The oil should be a beautiful golden color.

As it cools, the oil might thicken slightly, but it should remain liquid at room temperature. Discard the milk solids (or use them in your cooking).

Cautionary Note: If butter has been heated with aromatic essences, discard milk solids and *never* cook with them.

GHEE RECIPES

For incense purposes, all ghee is scented. Unscented, it will smell like butter. If you wish to store it for long periods of time, adding an anti-oxidant helps prevent rancidity. Liquid vitamin E drops work nicely.

JASMINE GHEE

1 pound butter
2 drops jasmine oil
2 drops vitamin E

Clarify the butter, and pour the oil into a jar. Add vitamin E to the oil after it has cooled, then add jasmine oil. Shake vigorously to blend oils uniformly. Pour ghee into a tightly covered jar for storage, or into your ghee lamp, saving the rest. Like any oil, ghee should be stored in a cool, dark location. It keeps best with refrigeration.

SANDALWOOD GHEE

1 pound butter
1 ounce sandalwood powder
2 drops vitamin E

Heat butter and sandalwood powder in pan. Clarify butter, and pour the oil into a jar. After it has cooled, add vitamin E.

LAVENDER GHEE

1 pound butter
1 ounce lavender flowers
2 drops vitamin E

Heat butter and lavender flowers. Clarify butter, adding vitamin E after the oil has cooled. Shake well and store in a cool, dry location.

FRANKINCENSE GHEE

1 pound butter
1 ounce powdered frankincense
2 drops vitamin E

Heat butter and frankincense. Clarify butter. Add vitamin E after oil has cooled. Shake well. Store in a cool, dry location.

Part 4

Colognes
&
Soaps

Chapter 11

European Colognes

EAU DE COLOGNE, the world famous toilet water, originated in the city of Cologne, (Köln) Germany, from whence it gets its name. The use of colognes quickly spread among the Royal families of Europe.

Early colognes were rather primitive, consisting of water perfumed by flowers. Pans of water filled with flower petals were set out in the sun. Towards evening, the pans were brought in, and the scented water was poured off into jars. The water had some of the fragrance of the flowers because the floral oils had seeped into it. Often some color seeped into the water as well, giving it a tint.

Today's colognes include alcohol and a fixative agent, usually in the form of glycerin. Glycerin works well because it is a liquid. You can use other fixing agents, such as benzoin gum or orris root, but, sometimes these powders don't entirely dissolve and settlings occur at the bottom of the container. This is undesirable from an aesthetic point of view.

COLOGNE COMPONENTS

Every cologne has four essential parts.

Water. Use only distilled water. Tap water can contain impurities, which can interfere with the aesthetics and aromatic qualities of a cologne.

Alcohol. Alcohol provides a solvent for the other ingredients. It also releases fragrances as it evaporates.

Fragrance. Floral oils, essential herbal oils, liquid gums, and resins can be used to provide fragrance, as can flower petals, herbal leaves, roots, and powders.

Fixing Agent. Various gums and resins can serve as a fixing agent to maintain the aromatic integrity of your colognes. Without a fixing agent the fragrance rapidly dissipates. Glycerin is an excellent fixative for colognes, as it is already a liquid and blends easily with other liquids.

Use of Flower Petals

If you use natural flower petals, herbs, roots, or leaves to scent your colognes, you'll need to remove the solid objects before the cologne is bottled, primarily for aesthetic reasons.

Some of the coloring pigments that occur naturally in the flowers or herbs will seep into the cologne. When using floral oils or essential herbal oils, you might wish to add an herbal colorant for aesthetic reasons. If you don't object to chemical colorants, use common food dyes for this purpose.

TRADITIONAL COLOGNE FROM FLOWERS

You can use several methods to prepare colognes from flowers. The first method is perhaps the oldest. Using crockery or a quart Mason jar, fill the jar with rose petals , packing them in tightly. Add distilled water to the jar until it is 3/4 full, then add two tablespoons of liquid vegetable oil. (Avoid highly scented oils, such as peanut oil, as they will interfere with your cologne. You probably don't want your cologne to smell like fresh peanuts, do you?) Finally, add 1 ounce of alcohol. Unscented rubbing alcohol works nicely.

Cover the jar with a tight lid. Shake contents thoroughly. Set the jar in a place where it won't be disturbed for a couple of days, and shake the jar each morning and evening to agitate the ingredients and speed up the process.

As the rose petals become saturated with water, the cellular membranes burst. This releases essential oils as well as some of the coloring pigments. These floral oils escape into the water and cling to the vegetable oil. The alcohol acts as a solvent, dissolving the oils so that they mix with the water. Otherwise, oil and water do not mix.

Agitating the jar helps speed the process of dispersing the floral oils. Naturally, the longer the petals are in the water, the more of their floral oils will be released, up to the point of *cellular saturation* or the point of diminishing returns, where longer time periods prove futile because the membranes can release no more essential oils. In other words you get the same results from letting it set for a couple of days as you would from letting it set a month or longer, so there is no point in extending the settling period in false hopes of extracting more fragrance.

After a few days you can pour the liquid cologne into jars for storage and discard the solids. Some people like to use a filter to keep solids out of their colognes: Cheesecloth works nicely for this purpose. If you did not add a fixing agent when you mixed the other ingredients, do so now. Glycerin blends in nicely. Use it at the rate of one ounce glycerin per quart.

Toilet waters made without alcohol have to be shaken before each use because the oils and water will separate. All the fragrance and most of the color will be attracted to the oils. This is the reason that alcohol was added originally.

Alternate Method

Another method of making cologne from fresh flowers uses alcohol as the base, with the water added later. First, pack the jar full of rose or other flower petals. Fill the jar to 1/2 full with unscented (rubbing) alcohol, and 2 tablespoons vegetable oil. Cover tightly, and shake the contents. Let it set for a couple of days. Agitate the jar each morning and evening, or as often as you like. Be sure to agitate it some so that the flower petals that are in the top of the jar get thoroughly wet with alcohol. The alcohol will act as a solvent, dissolving the colorant and essential oils into the oil and alcohol.

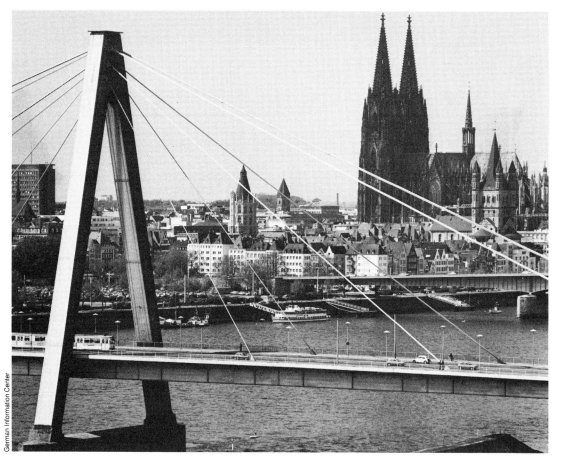

German Information Center

Cologne (Köln), Germany—the city that gave "eau de cologne" its name.

After a couple of days pour the mixture into other jars, and add water and glycerin at that time. Shake contents. You might wish to filter out solids so that your colognes sparkle. Don't forget to add water and glycerin or your cologne will rapidly evaporate and lose its aromatic qualities.

Fast Cologne

To speed up the process when making colognes from fresh flowers, simply place the jar in a sunny window. A hot afternoon can do the work of time. You will be able to see the petals' cellular breakdown and release of essential oils. By using this method you can often have cologne the same day, rather than waiting for a couple of days. Be sure the jar is kept tightly covered. Also, agitate it from time to time to help speed up the process dispersing the essential oils.

RECIPES

The colognes of each country tend to reflect the special scents that are part of each locale, since many colognes were originally made employing locally grown flowers and herbs. As trade between cities and nations increased, new fragrances were introduced.

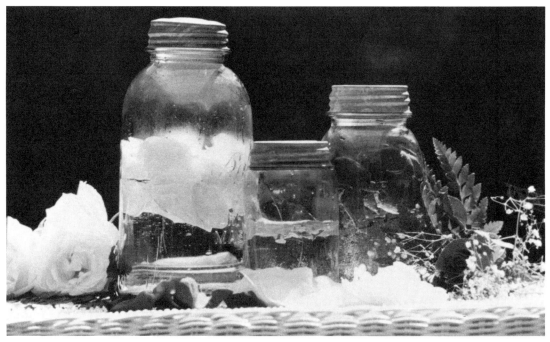

The traditional method of making cologne with flowers.

Rose colognes are universally popular. This is not surprising, since roses grow practically everywhere. The English are especially fond of lavender, and the French favor jasmine.

The following recipes are based on old European standards. Glycerin is used as the fixing agent for most because of its practicality. Also, herbs are substituted for animal oils, and English standards are used for measurements.

TRADITIONAL ROSE EAU DE COLOGNE

1 pint distilled water
4 ounces alcohol
1 ounce glycerin
1 drop rose geranium oil
1 drop rose oil
1 drop oil of bergamot

A colorant is optional. The same herbal colorants described in chapter 9 may be employed here. Add colorants as a liquid by preparing them with alcohol in a separate bowl—1 or 2 teaspoons of colorant powder to 1 teaspoon of alcohol. Usually just a few drops will provide the color you desire for your colognes.

Chemical colorants may be employed by those who do not object to their usage. Food-grade dyes available at most supermarkets work nicely.

ROYAL JASMINE COLOGNE

1 pint distilled water
1 ounce glycerin
4 ounces alcohol
1 teaspoon vanilla
1/4 teaspoon cinnamon
2 drops jasmine oil
1 drop bergamot oil
2 drops goldenrod tincture (colorant)

ROYAL SWEDISH COLOGNE

1 pint distilled water
1/4 pint alcohol
1 ounce glycerin
1 drop rose oil
2 drops violet oil
1 drop lemon oil
1 drop tonka bean extract
2 drops indigo tincture (colorant)

FLEUR D'COEUR COLOGNE

1 pint distilled water
4 ounces alcohol
1 ounce glycerin
1 drop rose oil
1 drop violet oil
1 drop gardenia oil
2 drops madder root tincture (colorant)

ENGLISH LAVENDER COLOGNE

1 pint distilled water
4 ounces alcohol
1 ounce glycerin
1 drop bergamot oil
2 drops lavender oil
2 drops black malva flowers tincture (colorant)

VICTORIAN LAVENDER COLOGNE

1 pint distilled water
4 ounces alcohol
1 ounce glycerin
1 drop rose oil
2 drops lavender oil
1 drop lemon oil
2 drops indigo tincture (colorant)

FRENCH LAVENDER COLOGNE

1 pint distilled water
4 ounces alcohol
1 ounce glycerin
2 teaspoons cinnamon
2 drops lavender oil
1 drop lemon oil
2 drop black malva flowers tincture (colorant)

SPANISH VALENCIA COLOGNE

1 pint distilled water
4 ounces alcohol
1 ounce glycerin
2 drops orange oil
1 drop lemon oil
2 drops annatto seed tincture (colorant)

SCOT COLOGNE

1 drop oil of bergamot
2 drops deer's tongue herbal extract
1 ounce glycerin
1 pint distilled water
4 ounces alcohol
2 drops goldenrod tincture (optional colorant)

ROYAL ENGLISH LAVENDER COLOGNE

1 pint distilled water
1 ounce glycerin
1 drop rose oil
1 drop bergamot oil
2 drops lavender
4 ounces alcohol
2 drops black malva flowers tincture (colorant)

HOUSE OF LANCASTER COLOGNE

1/4 pint alcohol
1 pint water
1 ounce glycerin
2 drops rose oil (Red Rose of Lancaster)
1 drop lemon oil
2 drops madder root tincture (colorant)

HOUSE OF YORK COLOGNE

1/4 pint alcohol
1 pint distilled water
1 ounce glycerin
2 drops rose oil (White Rose of York)
1 drop bergamot oil
1 teaspoon vanilla

COURT OF SAINT BRICE COLOGNE

1/4 pint alcohol
1 pint distilled water
1 ounce powdered frankincense (fixative)
1 drop rose oil
2 drops lilac oil
2 drops black malva flowers tincture (colorant)

SWEDISH VIOLET COLOGNE

$1/4$ pint alcohol
1 ounce glycerin
1 pint distilled water
1 drop deer's tongue herbal extract
1 drop rosemary oil
2 drops violet oil
2 drops indigo tincture (colorant)

Chapter 12

Oriental Colognes

ONE OF THE EXCITING things about the Orient is the way it enchants the five senses: sight, touch, taste, sound, and smell. The exotic fragrances of the Orient seem to linger, especially on the mind, perhaps because aromatic essences are an old art form and the Eastern cultures have existed for thousands of years. Whatever the reason, Eastern use of aromatic blends is exquisite, even spellbinding.

From Bombay to Xi'an to Hiroshima, the Orient offers a wealth of aromas. Some scents seem to conjure up images of grand pagodas, or hindu temples. India, Tibet, China, Mongolia, and Japan are among the special places of interest in the vast Asian continent.

INDIA

India has a large population—over 800 million people. In the next century, its population is expected to rise to over a billion and a half, outpacing China's population by a couple of hundred millions.

Although modern India has technology and industries not unlike most civilized nations, it still has a disproportionate number of its citizenry employed in agriculture. And, to its good fortune, village crafts still abound. Many of the skills the villagers have are similar to those our ancestors knew during the formative years of our country. Most of the skills these people have developed were handed down from the previous generation, and some are practically lost arts—one of the tragic consequences of progress. Fortunately, there has been a renewal of interest world-wide in many of these crafts.

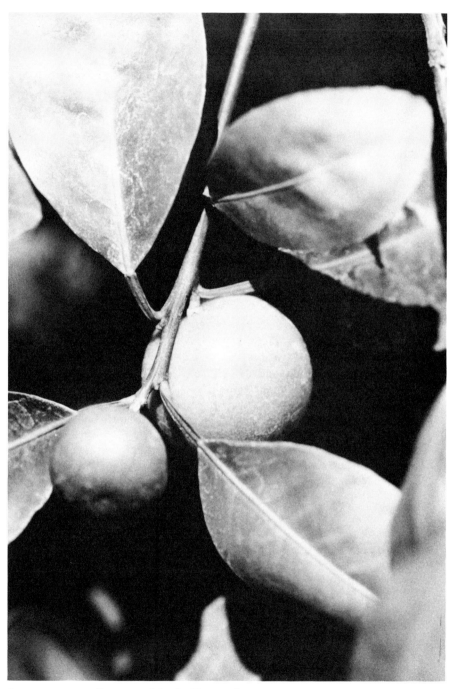

Lemons are often used in Indian colognes.

Much of the Indian subcontinent is characterized by subtropical *flora*, or plant life. In the mountainous north grow temperate-zone plants. If you climb up into the Himalayas that frame India's borders, you can even find plants that grow in the Arctic, so a wide variety of plant life characterizes the Indian subcontinent.

This is important to remember because it explains the wide range of fragrances that come out of India. Of course, trade has always spread the different aromatic essences. However, it is historically accurate to say that people usually use those plants native to their region primarily and most abundantly, which is true even today. If a flower grows in your backyard, you are more likely to use it than if it grows only in Hawaii some 4,000 miles away!

When you realize the importance of proximity of ingredients, it's easy to understand why Indian colognes are so abundant in their employment of fragrant woods, gums, resins, and spices.

Indian Colognes

TAJ MAHAL COLOGNE

1/4 pint alcohol
1 pint distilled water
1 ounce sandalwood powder (fixative)
1 teaspoon tonka bean extract
1/4 teaspoon cinnamon
1 drop oleander oil
1 drop lemon oil
2 drops saffron tincture (colorant)

BOMBAY COLOGNE

1/4 pint alcohol
1 pint distilled water
1 ounce sandalwood powder (fixative)
1 drop patchouli oil
1 drop lemon oil
1/4 teaspoon cinnamon

CALCUTTA COLOGNE

1 pint distilled water
1/4 pint alcohol
1 ounce powdered frankincense (fixative)
1 teaspoon nutmeg
1 teaspoon cinnamon
1 drop tonka bean extract
1 drop lemon oil

SANDALWOOD COLOGNE

1 pint distilled water
4 ounces alcohol
1 ounce glycerin
1/4 teaspoon cinnamon
2 drops sandalwood
1 drop lemon oil

SONG OF INDIA COLOGNE

1 pint distilled water
4 ounces alcohol
1 ounce sandalwood powder (fixative)
1 tablespoon powdered myrrh gum
1 tablespoon powdered frankincense gum
1 drop patchouli oil
1 drop tonka bean extract
1/4 teaspoon nutmeg
1/2 teaspoon cinnamon

SRI LANKA CINNAMON COLOGNE

1/4 pint alcohol
1 ounce glycerin
1 pint distilled water
1 teaspoon vanilla
1 drop cinnamon oil
1 drop lemon oil

TIBET

High up in the Himalayan Mountains lies the land of Shangri La, known as Tibet. Today it is a province of the People's Republic of China. The people are predominantly of Mongoloid stock. Modified racial types, a product of intermarriage between Chinese and Indian peoples, are common in the frontier regions and in large cities.

Most of the people belong to a religious sect called Lamaism, with its spiritual leader, the "Dali Lama."

Vegetation is sparse in many of the plateau regions, while along the river valleys, temperate zone plants—such as apples, peaches, and apricots—thrive.

Because it is surrounded by mountains, Tibet has enjoyed a certain isolation from much of the outside world. Village crafts and ancient customs are still found throughout the nation.

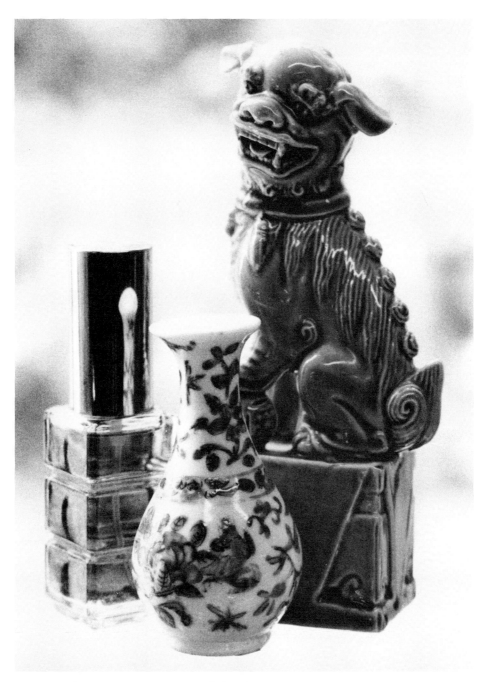

Exotic colognes reminiscent of the Orient.

Tibetan Colognes

TIBET MUSK COLOGNE

1 pint distilled water
1/4 pint alcohol
1 ounce glycerin
1 drop cedar oil
2 drops synthetic musk oil

LAMA MONK COLOGNE

1/4 pint alcohol
1 pint distilled water
1 ounce gylcerin
1 drop patchouli oil
2 drops synthetic musk oil

Musk oil is a favorite component of most Tibetan colognes. Synthetic musk oil is a good substitute for people who object to use of animal extracts.

TIBETAN PEACH COLOGNE

1 pint distilled water
4 ounces alcohol (peach liquor)
1 ounce sandalwood powder (fixative)
1 drop rose oil
1 drop synthetic musk oil

TIBETAN APPLE COLOGNE

1 pint apple jack (hard cider)
1/2 pint distilled water
1 ounce powdered benzoin gum
1 teaspoon cinnamon
1/4 teaspoon nutmeg
1 drop synthetic musk oil

TIBETAN APRICOT COLOGNE

1 pint distilled water
1/2 pint apricot brandy
1 ounce glycerin
1 drop synthetic musk oil
1/2 teaspoon nutmeg

HIMALAYAN COLOGNE

1/4 pint alcohol
1 ounce glycerin
1 pint distilled water
1 drop patchouli oil
1 drop bergamot oil
1 drop synthetic musk oil

CHINA

The world's most populous nation is the People's Republic of China, which includes the province of Tibet. China is also one of the oldest ongoing societies in the world. It was a cradle of civilization.

The Chinese take great pride in their history and rightly so—few nations are as rich in history as is China. The Chinese people are industrious and place a high value on education. Under the late Mao ZeDong, hunger was eliminated in China.

China has a temperate climate for the most part, although its exterior has extremes of hot and cold, and the southern tip has subtropical flora. Most of the population lives in the eastern half of the nation. The deserts and barren plateaus of the west are not the most habitable of places, although nomadic tribes once inhabited those areas. Today most of the descendants of the nomadic tribes live in permanent settlements.

Chinese Colognes

CHINA ROSE COLOGNE

1 pint distilled water
4 ounces alcohol
1 ounce glycerin
1 teaspoon cinnamon
2 drops rose oil (China rose)

CHINA TEA ROSE COLOGNE

1/4 pint alcohol
1 pint water
1 ounce glycerin
2 drops rose oil (Tea rose)
1 drop lemon oil

HANGZHOU COLOGNE

1 pint distilled water
4 ounces cherry brandy
1 ounce glycerin
2 drops ylang ylang oil
1 drop rose oil

QIATANG RIVER COLOGNE

1 pint distilled water
2 ounces peach brandy
2 ounces cherry brandy
1 ounce glycerin
1 drop tonka bean extract
2 drops oleander oil

SHANGHAI COLOGNE

1 pint distilled water
4 ounces alcohol
2 teaspoons nutmeg
1 ounce glycerin
1 drop heliotrope oil
1 drop oleander oil

HONG KONG COLOGNE

1/4 pint alcohol
1 ounce glycerin
1 drop wisteria oil
1 drop rose oil
1 drop lemon oil
1 teaspoon vanilla

KONG FOREST COLOGNE

1/4 pint alcohol
1 pint distilled water
1 ounce glycerin
1 drop pine needle oil
2 teaspoons sandalwood powder
1 teaspoon cedar powder
1 drop rose oil
1 drop oil of bergamot
1 drop violet oil

MONGOLIA

Mongolia is home to the once nomadic Mongol tribes, although many Mongols and their descendants are scattered all over the world. The modern nation of Mongolia consists of an area called Outer Mongolia. The region known as Inner Mongolia is part of China.

The Mongols are most famous as ancient warriors. Ghengis Khan is a name recognized even today, but Mongolia reached its zenith under his son, Kublai Khan, who ruled China. Marco Polo was a guest of the Court of Kublai Khan.

Mongolian Colognes

COURT OF KUBLAI KHAN COLOGNE

1/4 pint alcohol
1 pint distilled water
1 ounce glycerin
1 drop wisteria oil
1 drop rose oil
1 drop bergamot oil
1 drop synthetic musk oil

MONGOLIAN COLOGNE

1 pint distilled water
1/4 pint alcohol
1 ounce glycerin
1 drop bergamot oil
2 drops synthetic musk oil

JAPAN

The Japanese Islands stretch along the northern rim of Asia. For many centuries Japan lived in physical isolation from its neighbors. Occasionally, there were skirmishes with Korea, and sometimes with China, too. Later, after the introduction of western technology, Japan became a major world power.

Japanese Colognes

TOKYO ROSE COLOGNE

1 pint distilled water
4 ounces cherry brandy
1 ounce glycerin
2 drops rose oil
1 drop lemon oil
1 drop synthetic musk oil

ROYAL NIPPON COLOGNE

1 pint distilled water
1/4 cherry alcohol
1 drop carnation oil
1 drop oleander oil
1 drop rose oil
1 drop synthetic musk oil
1 teaspoon vanilla

Note: The majority of the cologne recipes in this chapter have been prepared without the addition of colorants. If you wish to use a coloring agent, do so as instructed in chapter 10. Herbal colorants are listed in chapter 9, and chemical colorants are available at your local supermarket. Remember that only a couple of drops of colorant are all that is usually needed.

Chapter 13

Soap

THE ART OF MAKING SOAP is an ancient craft. The cleansing agents mentioned in the Old Testament were not true soaps, but were made from wood ashes. During the first century A.D., the Roman historian Pliny mentioned various hard and soft soaps used in Rome. By the eighth century A.D., soap making was common in Italy and Spain.

By the thirteenth century, soap making was introduced into France. The French experimented and developed a method of making soap from olive oil. Prior to that time, goat tallow was the fat used most frequently, and the ashes of beechwood provided the alkali. This soap was introduced into England around 1500 as Castile soap. Presumably it got that name because the olive oil used to make it had come from the Kingdom of Castile (part of modern-day Spain).

In 1783 the Swedish chemist, Karl Wilhem Scheele, discovered glycerin. But it wasn't until 1823 that French chemist Michel Eugene Chevreul discovered that fats do not combine with alkali to form soap, but first are decomposed into fatty acids and glycerols.

In 1791 French chemist Nicholas LeBlanc invented a process to obtain lye from ordinary salt.

In the early days of the United States, most soap was made at home from rendered animal fats and wood ashes. It remained a household product for many decades. As early as 1700, however, some people made a profitable business out of selling fats and ashes to be used in home soap making. Instead of purchasing ready-made soap as we do today, some colonials—especially those who lived in urban areas and didn't have access to animals or wood—would buy the ingredients from various tradesmen and make their own soap at home.

HOMEMADE SOAP

Three ingredients are essential to making soap—fats, alkali, and water.

131

FATS—Vegetable oils; also tallow and fish oils for those who do not object to using animal fats.
ALKALI—Lye, either caustic soda or potassium hydroxide, or wood ashes.
WATER

All other ingredients are added for a specific purpose, to modify the soap. For example, some ingredients are added as emollients to make soap gentle to the skin. Others are added for fragrance or to give soap color. Soap that is made without the addition of emollients is likely to be too harsh to the skin for daily use. It is better suited to laundry purposes.

Emollients

Any number of different ingredients are added to soap to make it less harsh. All fall under the broad category of *emollients*. These can include vitamins A, C, D, and E, and sometimes panthenol and/or para-amino-benezoic acid (PABA).

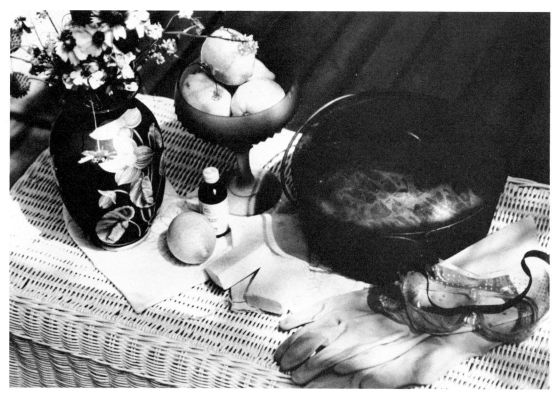

Some of the tools and ingredients you'll need to make soap.

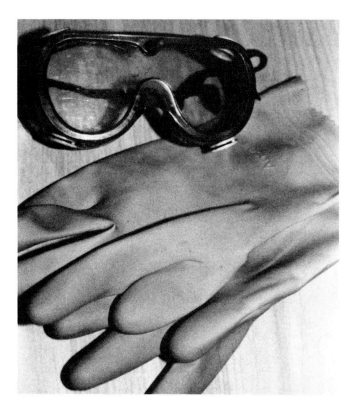

Always wear goggles and rubber gloves for protection when making soap.

Various oils may also be added to soap as emollients for the skin. Cocoa butter is a favorite, as is lanolin, which is extracted from the wool of sheep. Aloe vera gel is another popular ingredient. Aloe vera was used by Cleopatra as a beauty aid. Other emollients are jojoba oil and coconut oil. The latter is popular in soap because it makes for a rich lather. Other oils that make good soaps include castor oil, peach kernel oil, wheat germ oil, and many more.

Never add ingredients that are poisonous, or that you are allergic to. If you are offering your homemade soaps for sale, be sure that they have enough emollients in them to be extra gentle to the skin. Customers might hold you liable if they develop an allergic rash or if the soap is too harsh for personal use.

HOW TO MAKE SOAP

The first thing you'll want to do once you have decided to make a batch of soap is to get ready for the project. You must have all the equipment that you need on hand. Wear long-sleeved shirts, trousers not shorts, and rubber gloves. Put on safety eye goggles.

Once you have dressed for safety, check to see that you have all ingredients within easy reach so you won't forget something at the last minute or waste time looking for something while your soap scorches on the stove. Careful preparation is the best way to begin any project, and it is vital when making soap. If you have everything where it is out and convenient, you will be less likely to run into any snafus.

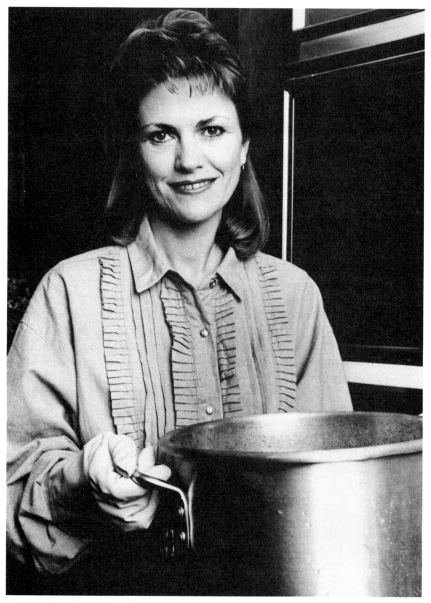

Large kettles work best for soap making.

Soap making is not an activity for small children. It must be done in a well-ventilated room free of distractions. You cannot watch television and make soap at the same time. If you have a favorite program on television, plan your soap making project for afterwards so you will be able to concentrate entirely on the project at hand. Put aside a special time when you will be able to make your soap without any outside distractions. Don't make soap if you're upset, worried, or depressed. You will need your full attention to the task at hand.

Always allow yourself enough time to do the job right. Soap is not something you can leave half-finished; you have to do the job from start to finish. With careful preparation, you should be able to make a batch of soap within one hour.

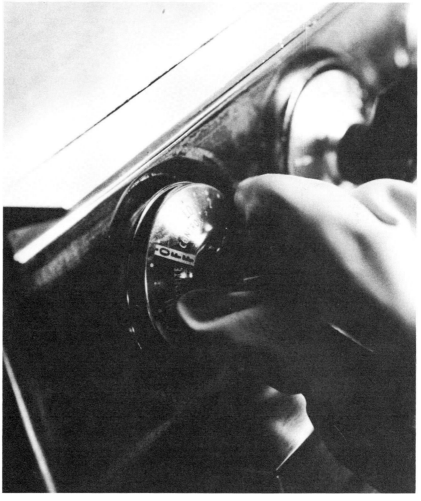

Heat at a low setting.

Keep pets, kids, and friends out of the area; they can distract you or get injured. *Always* wear eye goggles when making soap. Lye is a caustic substance and must be handled with extreme care. Also, the fumes given off by the saponification process can cause blindness, so protect your eyes!

Important Things to Remember

Whenever you are involved in making soap, always follow directions carefully. You really cannot expect to achieve decent results if you skim over instructions and do things "by guess and by gosh."

Secondly, always handle materials with care. Add lye to *cold* water only. Never under any circumstance should you add lye to hot water! Reread the preceding sentence until you have committed it to memory. Carelessness in handling lye can result in severe burns or blindness.

Third, if you are trying to make soap as the pioneers and colonials did—with wood ashes—be sure that the ashes are *only* wood. Do not use coal ashes or those from charcoal briquettes: These can contain chemicals that irritate your skin. The colonials used ashes from hardwood trees, such as oak. Sift the ashes, and use only the fine powdery ashes. You do not want chunks of charcoal or small pieces of half-burned wood in your soap.

Once you have your equipment in place and are wearing clothes that will protect you from accidental splashes or spills, put on your safety goggles. At the risk of sounding redundant, the importance of wearing protective clothing cannot be stressed enough. Soap gets very hot and can cause severe burns.

Do you have all your ingredients? The emollients that you will be adding? Colorant? Have a checklist if need be so that you can check off ingredients as you use them. You are now ready to begin.

HARD SOAP RECIPES

Hard soap, or bar soap, is the kind of soap most people think of when they talk about soap. All hard soap is made with *caustic soda* or *sodium hydroxide* (lye). Lye is available at many supermarkets.

Can Instructions

Often the can of lye you purchase will have instructions for its use in making soap printed right on its back label. Follow those instructions, even if you wish to improvise your own recipe, or follow a recipe in this book. For example, the amount of water you add to a recipe can vary—sometimes different manufacturers recommend different amounts. This is where you need to employ common sense and personal discretion. Water acts only as a solvent for the lye and to facilitate saponification. Any "excess" water only prolongs the time it takes for the mixture to become soap.

Cooking Instructions

Place the cold water in a large kettle on the stove. Stir the lye into the cold water until it dissolves. Add the shortening, and stir it a couple of times.

Turn the stove on. Cook at a low to medium setting, stirring continuously with a large *wooden* spoon. Stir slowly so you don't splash any of the mixture.

Saponification takes place as the mixture thickens and spits up like gravy. Once saponification occurs, remove from the heat. As the soap starts to cool, but before it has hardened, add whatever emollients you wish and blend them in thoroughly. Add a colorant, if you desire, after you have added all the emollients. As a final step, add whatever fragrance you want. *Never* add fragrance while the soap is hot: Add it just before pouring the soap into molds.

LEMON SOAP

1 pound shortening (hydrogenated)
4 ounces lye dissolved in 8 ounces cold water
2 ounces aloe vera
1 ounce coconut oil
3 drops lemon oil
2 drops saffron tincture (colorant)

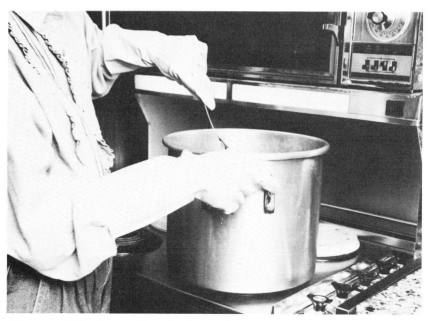

Stir carefully to avoid splashing the hot mixture.

VITAMIN E SOAP

1 pound hydrogenated vegetable shortening
1/4 pound lye, dissolved in 8 ounces cold water
1 ounce glycerin
1 ounce lanolin
2 tablespoons coconut oil
1 ounce vitamin E liquid

ENGLISH LAVENDER SOAP

1 pound shortening
4 ounces lye, dissolved in 8 ounces cold water
1 ounce glycerin
1 ounce cocoa butter
2 drops lavender oil
1 drop rose oil
1 drop lemon oil
2 drops black malva flowers tincture (colorant)

ROSE SOAP

1 pound shortening
4 ounces lye
8 ounces cold water
1 ounce coconut oil
1 ounce aloe vera gel
2 drops rose oil
1 drop lemon oil
2 drops madder root tincture (colorant)

SRI LANKA CINNAMON SOAP

1 pound shortening
4 ounces lye, dissolved in 8 ounces cold water
2 ounces lanolin
1 ounce coconut oil
3 tablespoons cinnamon
2 drops henna tincture (colorant)

TIBETAN MUSK SOAP

1 pound shortening
4 ounces lye
8 ounces cold water
2 ounces lanolin
3 drops synthetic musk oil
2 drops catechu tincture (colorant)

INDIAN SANDALWOOD SOAP

1 pound shortening
4 ounces lye
8 ounces cold water
2 ounces powdered sandalwood
1 teaspoon cinnamon
1 ounce coconut oil
1 ounce glycerin
2 drops butternut tincture (colorant)

ALOE VERA SOAP

1 pound shortening
4 ounces lye
8 ounces cold water
3 ounces aloe vera gel
1 ounce glycerin
2 drops almond oil
2 drops goldenrod tincture (colorant)

LANOLIN SOAP

1 pound shortening
4 ounces lye, dissolved in 8 ounces cold water
4 ounces lanolin
1 drop almond oil
1 drop lemon oil
2 drops saffron tincture (colorant)

OATMEAL SOAP

1 pound shortening
4 ounces lye
8 ounces cold water
2 ounces aloe vera
1 ounce glycerin
1 ounce cocoa butter
2 teaspoons vanilla

CASTILE SOAP

16 ounces virgin olive oil
4 ounces lye
8 ounces cold water
2 ounces lanolin
2 drops almond oil

ROYAL VERSAILLES SOAP

16 ounces virgin olive oil
4 ounces powdered wood ash or lye dissolved in 8 ounces cold water
3 ounces lanolin
1 drop rose oil
2 drops violet oil
1 drop synthetic musk oil
2 drops indigo tincture (colorant)

ROYAL FRENCH JASMINE SOAP

16 ounces virgin olive oil
4 ounces lye
8 ounces cold water
3 ounces lanolin
1 ounce coconut oil
2 drops jasmine oil
2 drops goldenrod tincture (colorant)

LIQUID SOAP

Liquid soaps are made by using potassium hydroxide (lye) as the alkali agent. Check your can's label to be sure that the lye you are using is the right one for the job.

Liquid soap was once confined to public rest rooms. Today, its popularity has grown, and it can be found in households all across America.

LIQUID WHITE ROSE SOAP

1 pound hydrogenated vegetable shortening
4 onces potassium hydroxide (lye)
24 ounces cold water (3 cups)
2 ounces glycerine
2 ounces coconut oil
2 ounces aloe vera
3 drops rose oil
1 drop lemon oil

Place the water in a kettle on the stove. Add the lye (use potassium hydroxide) to the cold water, stirring it in so that it dissolves. Add the vegetable shortening. (You can substitute an equivalent amount of vegetable oil for shortening if you prefer, but remember: liquid vegetable oils will add color, whereas white hydrogenated shortening is necessary to give the finished product its white color without the addition of a colorant.)

Mix thoroughly, stirring carefully so it doesn't splash around. Turn on the stove to a low or medium flame. Continue to stir with a long-handled wooden spoon. (Never use a metal spoon; it will get too hot to handle.) The mixture has saponified (become soap) when the consistency is like a gravy and it is spitting up in the pan.

Remove the soap from heat. Carefully stir air into the mixture; it will thicken more as it cools. Add emollients before the soap has completely cooled, then add a colorant if desired. Add fragrance last. Stir to blend ingredients evenly. When the soap is cool, pour it into permanent containers or dispensers.

SOAP POWDER

Soap powder is made by grating a cake of hard soap. Although soap powders are used in some public rest rooms, historically they were used in laundry, especially before the invention of modern detergents.

You may add emollients to your laundry soap powders. If you spend much time with your hands in the wash basin or laundry tub, that might be a good idea. Otherwise, it isn't crucial. Most people do not add colorants to soap powders.

If soap powders are to be used for personal hygiene, such as in a rest room, it will be very important to add emollients to keep the soap from being too harsh for delicate skin.

The easiest way to make soap powder is by making your favorite bar recipe. The cakes or bars of soap can then be grated into a fine powder. For a sudsy laundry soap, use a recipe that includes coconut oil.

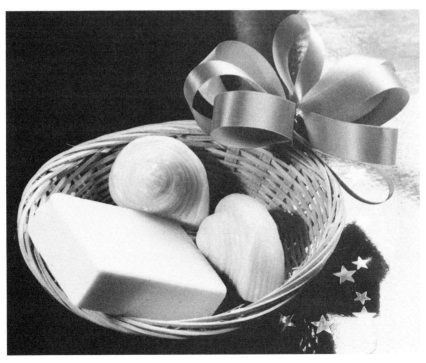

Display your homemade soap proudly.

Chapter 14

Unusual Soaps

SOAP MAKING IS AN OLD ART. The different peoples of the world have developed many unique and interesting customs, including the imaginative ways that they have turned soap making from a simple craft into an art.

TURKEY'S FRUIT-SHAPED SOAP

The Turkish city of Edirne has earned a distinguished place in Turkish culture because of an unusual handicraft—they make fruit-shaped soaps.

Craftspeople created fruit shapes from a soap paste. They didn't use a press or a mold. Once the paste was the desired shape, the soap was then painted and dried. A stem appropriate to its shape was attached. By their clever use of materials and craftsmanship, the Turks of Edirne turned a daily necessity item (soap) into a brilliant work of art.

As a handicraft, fruit-shaped soap making was once common in Edirne. Unfortunately the craft has almost died out, primarily for economic reasons. Although some of the elders still possess the special skills necessary, most of the young are more interested in making money (like young people everywhere), and the tradition is being lost.

Today no stores sell this fruit-shaped soap. The only place they are found is in museums, or among the private collections of wealthy investors who collect primitive art and crafts.

Amateurs who want to try making fruit-shaped soaps of their own might have to use some ingenuity rather than trying to reconstruct the Turkish method, unless you are fortunate enough to have access to their secrets. You can purchase fruit-shaped molds for this project, and these are the best bet for the neophyte. Molds provide the novice with an easy way to achieve the desired shapes without having the skill to construct them from scratch.

Pour the soap into the mold—a peach mold, for example's sake. To add to the illusion, you might want to use peach oil to scent the soap. After the peach-shaped soap has dried it will be ready for use. It can never compare with the soaps of Edirne as art, but it is suitable for the uses of most people.

SEASHELL SOAP

You can make special soaps by using seashell-shaped molds. The soap can be scented with whatever fragrance you desire, and you can add colorant to give it a peach or pink hue. Of course, colorants are always optional ingredients.

For variety you can use different sizes of shell molds. It is usually best to avoid molds that are extremely large because it will take longer for the soap to harden. Also, soap that doesn't fit in the palm of your hand is not as easy to use in washing.

Usually people make several bars from a batch. Sometimes they make several batches, adding different scents and/or colorants for effect.

ALTERNATIVES TO BAR SOAP

Soap can be molded into an unlimited variety of shapes and sizes. Ordinary cookie cutters can create interesting soaps, but it is important to

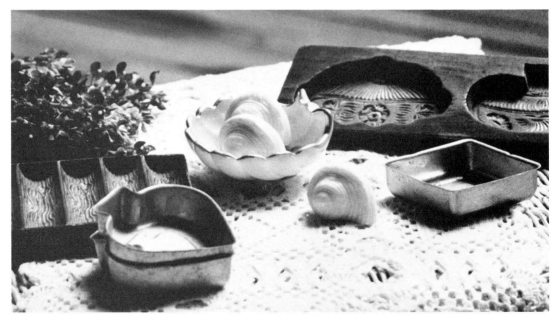

Most soaps are unusual because of their shapes.

use only sturdy molds. Avoid plastic because these molds can crack or melt if the soap is too hot.

A good source of molds for soap making can be found at many craft and hobby shops. Specialty molds can be ordered through mail order specialty craft companies. (See Appendix.)

Toy soldiers, cars, trains, and almost anything you can imagine are the various shapes to which soap has been molded. The clever entrepreneur will be able to master ideas of his or her own as well.

Soap on a Rope

Yarn is usually used to provide the rope for soap on a rope. Don't use real ropes made from hemp because these might be too hard on the hands, causing blisters.

Yarn is available in many bright or pastel colors. It is easily woven into ropes that are sturdy enough for the purpose of hanging soap.

Soap Rolls

Do you get upset because your soap dishes are always messy? Or have you ever wondered if there weren't some possible use of the multitude of empty toilet paper rolls you toss in the garbage (or your fireplace) regularly? Now you can combine the two problems and come up with one solution: soap rolls.

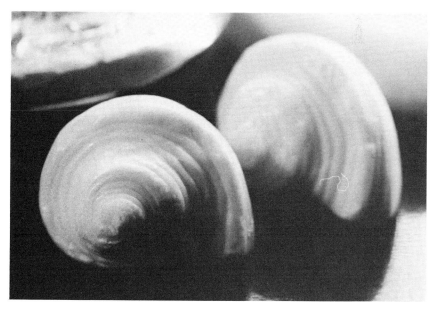

Seashell soap.

Save your empty toilet paper rolls as you use your toilet paper. When you have the desired quantity for a batch, use them to shape your very special soap into a unique gift for friends or a hot sales item for customers looking for something out of the ordinary.

To make soap rolls, you will need a wooden tray or cake pan lined with heavy paper. Place the toilet paper rolls upright, touching each other. At each side of the tray, place a block of wood or other object with sufficient weight to keep the rolls firmly in place when your pour in the hot soap (Remember to save the bits of soap that might cling to the bottom of the tray for your liquid soap.) Use your favorite hard soap recipe.

Soap Pockets

One problem that is universal in most households is what to do with the slivers of old soap that accumulate in the soap basin. Most people don't like washing with them because they are often small and awkward to use. They also have lost any aesthetic appeal they might have once had.

One way to make use of these slivers is to create soap pockets. To make soap pockets, simply sew together two washcloths at three ends. Place a zipper along the fourth border to make it easy to remove and refill the pockets. If you wish to sell the soap pockets as a novelty, you should include a fresh bar of soap. Customers might feel cheated if you fill them with old slivers of soap.

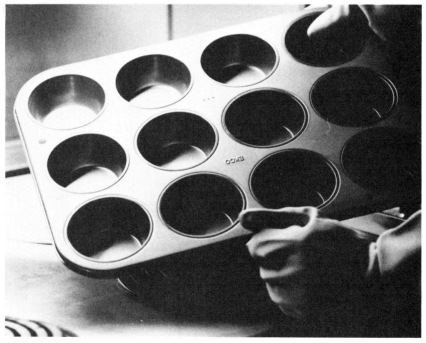

You can use an ordinary cupcake tin as a soap mold.

Always use clean washcloths. Although rags can be used as a substitute, select only those materials that will be soft and comfortable to wash with. Scratch fabrics or old underwear will never do. Brightly colored, new washcloths are most attractive. Some people like to embroider designs on soap pockets, but this actually makes it less comfortable to wash with.

For convenient storage and/or display, sew a handle onto the corner of each pocket to make it easy to hang up. Remember when you sew on the handle to place it where it will not interfere with the zipper. You must have access to the soap so that you can refill the pocket.

Soap Mittens

Soap mittens are another handy way to utilize old soap slivers. They are very similar to soap pockets, except they are in mitten form.

An easy way to make soap mittens is to sew a pocket onto an existing mitten's palm. Again, include a zipper so you can refill the mitt with soap.

Expert sewers may wish to make their own soap mittens from scratch. When making mittens for small children, remember to use small mittens that will fit tiny hands. An easy way to prevent feuds over whose mittens belong to whom is to give each child a separate color. Bright colors are usually more appealing to children than brown or gray colors.

When adding the soap pouch, select a material that complements the mitt so the pouch looks like an integral part of the mitten rather than shoddy patchwork. On the other hand, you might prefer the patchwork look. It's really up to you.

Part 5

Crafts for Today's Lifestyle

Chapter 15

Shortcuts

IN TODAY'S BUSY WORLD, time is an element that many people have in short supply. No matter how hard you try, you often find yourself with very little time to pursue the things that really interest you, or you're too busy to engage in a project that is time-consuming. For these and other reasons you want fast solutions.

There are several ways to do any project, and some methods are quicker and easier than others. A similar statement can be made about people: Some people have a knack for making simple chores difficult. It often is not the chore itself that is time-consuming, but rather the efficiency (or inefficiency) in the way you organize your time and materials. Being organized is a real secret to success in any project and makes it easier to complete in a shorter time.

POTPOURRI

Mixing up potpourri is easy and doesn't have to take much time. The following are some tricks that will help you save time:

- ✿ Gather all ingredients before you begin. This simple step is a real time-saver because much time is wasted in looking for ingredients as they are to be used in a recipe.
- ✿ Use ready-made containers. Much time is wasted in making containers. If you can select containers that are ready-made it will cut time.
- ✿ Purchase ready-made potpourri and add to it. It isn't exactly cheating. A ready-made potpourri can be personalized by adding your favorite scents. Often busy people will purchase potpourri and use it as a base, adding a few extra ingredients to their own liking. This is a fast and economical way of doing things and, by using a ready-made potpourri, you don't need to add a fixing agent. You often save on other ingredients, too.

151

Adding to a Mix

The important thing to keep in mind when adding to an existing pot-pourri is that the additives must not clash with the base. For example, if you want a rose potpourri, don't buy a cinnamon-apple potpourri to use as a base. It will not work to try to mask a potpourri. Any time you have to overcome one scent with another, you have already destroyed the delicate bouquet that is essential to a good potpourri.

The fragrances that you add must blend in or complement the pot-pourri. It never works to try to mask another odor: To do so will create a conflict of odors and everyone will ask, "What stinks?"

The following is a partial list of ingredients that can be added to a pot-pourri. It is *not* all-inclusive:

Apples, bananas, orange peel, lemon peel, tangerine peel, lime peel, grapefruit peel. Pineapple, grapes, strawberries, red raspberries. Peaches, apricots.

Allspice, cinnamon, nutmeg, cloves, ginger, anise, cardamon, paprika. Sweet basil, bay leaves, bayberry, caraway, celery, dill, fennel. Parsley, sage, rosemary, thyme. Damiana, dragon's blood, deer's tongue, savory, tarragon, catnip. Vanilla, tonka bean, coumarin, sweet fern, fenu-greek, gentian, horehound. Hyssop, licorice, liverwort, marigold, mullein, nettle, oregano, red clover. Plaintain, saffron, scullcap, yarrow. Sassafrass, sasparilla.

Peppermint, spearmint, applemint, wintergreen. Rose, lilac, lavender, violet, gardenia, heliotrope, lily-of-the-valley, sweet pea, wisteria, olean-der, verbena, ylang ylang, carnation, honeysuckle.

Sandalwood, cedar, pine needles, balsam fir, birch. And many, many more!

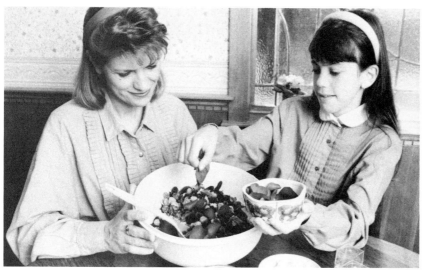

Quick recipes help working moms.

152

SOAP

Instant liquid soap is very easy to make. Gather up those small scraps and slivers of old soap bars—you know, the pieces nobody likes to use anymore. Keep them in a quart Mason jar and add water. You might want to add a tablespoon of coconut oil for lather and a drop of almond oil or whatever scent for fragrance.

Cover the jar with a tight lid. Shake it and let it set overnight. Shake it again. If you are in a hurry you will be able to use it without letting it set, but you must shake it first each time or the soap will settle to the bottom.

You can make hard soap fast from leftover slivers of soap. Gather them up and place them in a spot where the pieces will dry, or heat them in the oven at low heat for a few minutes to get them to dry. Once they are dry, grate the pieces into powder. Use your eyedropper to add a drop or two of water—not too much—just enough to form a paste. Put soap in a mold, and stick it in the refrigerator to quicken its hardening. The soap will be ready to use when it is firm.

READY-MADE CONTAINERS

Packaging has a visual impact on people. This is especially true in sales but packaging also affects everyone because it creates a visual image of the fragrances in our minds.

By selecting containers that harmonize with the fragrances of our potpourris, we create the total effect of the product. For example, if you have a strawberry potpourri, don't put it in a blue ceramic jar or a purple one. Select a container that will let people understand that it is a strawberry potpourri. Red or other colors associated with strawberries would be favored. The same can be said of other types of potpourri and sachets.

Fancy, ready-to-use packagings are available at many stores, or they can be custom made by a friend or from a specialty firm. These offer quick solutions to the busy person who simply doesn't have the time to make their own containers.

ENLISTING OTHERS

Some families who are short on friends and/or extended family often reach out to others in the community, especially the elderly. Many elderly people have time on their hands and not enough activities to fill it. A great number of these people might have developed special skills over their lifetimes. By getting in touch with these people you can enjoy the advantage of their time and talents enlisted for your projects.

A good place to locate talented elderly people is through senior citizen centers. Often a large number of people are anxious to help. Sometimes you can locate such people by asking your minister or priest about people in your church who might like to help you.

You might be surprised at how many elderly people there are who are more than delighted to help you with your home crafts, and for free!

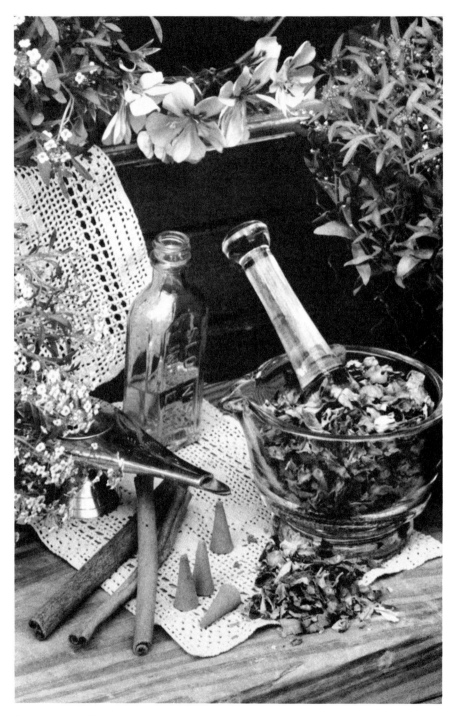

Only you will know you made it in a snap!

Chapter 16

Marketing Your Homemade Crafts

THERE IS ALWAYS A MARKET for homemade crafts. Finding one should not be that difficult for you. The problem that most people encounter is in choosing which is the best market for them. You'll need to consider many factors, including your inclinations and temperament.

RETAIL

Your personality is important because it can have a pivotal role in your success. For example, someone who tends to be hotheaded would be better in wholesale sales rather than retail sales. Jobbers (wholesalers) don't often meet with the general public. They do the bulk of their business with retailers. Only ordinary business skills are necessary when they are dealing with people in the industry.

The general public, however, is a very different matter. People can be rude, vulgar, and verbally abusive and still expect you to respond cheerfully and try to satisfy their every whim. There are people out there who have apparently never heard of mouthwash or deodorant. It is perhaps an understatement to suggest that any time you do business with the general public, you are in for an educational experience.

While it might be true that most people appear to be civil, you'd be surprised at what a short fuse your customers can have. The moment they can't find exactly what they want, they might react in anger. The public can also be fickle. They complain if nobody greets them to wait on them, and they also complain if you wait on them too eagerly. They ask you for suggestions and argue with you when you give them. The important thing to remember is that even if people ask you for your opinion, they often don't want *your* opinion. What they want is someone who will confirm their opinions, however bizarre those opinions might be.

Customers sometimes purchase a product only to return it later complaining that it wasn't what they wanted. Customers might lecture you about having high prices on your items; on the other hand, they won't buy something that is marked too cheap, perhaps reasoning, that if something is any good it has to cost money.

All this and more contradictory behavior you can expect from dealing with the general public. Some people take offense easily. What you might consider a harmless joke, another will react to as if it were holy blasphemy.

Anyone who is hot tempered isn't likely to enjoy working with the general public. Ordinary people can exhibit weird behavior. But customers have one big advantage over you: You need them a whole lot more than they need you. You might have to put up with nonsense in order to make a sale and keep the sales coming. Even more important to a business than making that first sale is getting repeat business, and the only way to have steady customers is if you make them feel special.

Desirable Traits

The most important traits you'll need to make it in retail sales are:

- ✿ Patience.
- ✿ Willingness to listen sympathetically.
- ✿ Friendliness. Everybody likes to be liked. People with friendly ways attract customers to your store and sell merchandise.
- ✿ Readiness to smile. More products are sold through a smile than by anything else.

Undesirable Traits

The best way to fail in a business is to exhibit any or all of these undesirable traits:

- ✿ Hotheadedness. As a salesperson you have to keep your cool at all times, even (and especially) when a customer becomes verbally abusive.
- ✿ Argumentativeness. The old adage applies in business, "The customer is always right." Even when they are clearly in the wrong, you are in business to sell merchandise to people, not to debate them. And don't think that you can really win an argument. For even if you prove yourself to be correct, you might lose a customer in the process. It's a no-win situation.
- ✿ Rudeness. Rudeness is never appropriate to business and always hurts sales.
- ✿ Bigotry. Prejudice is bad business.

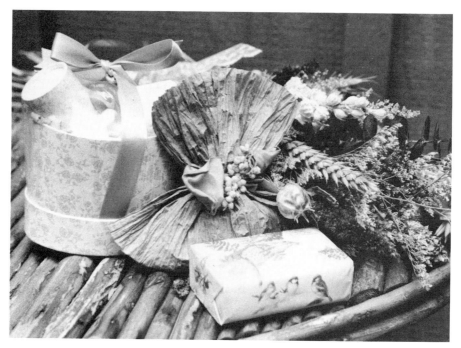

Display your wares attractively.

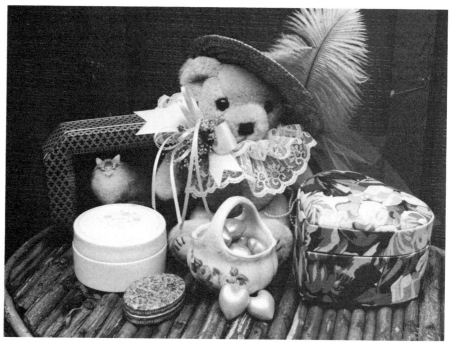

There is always a market for homemade crafts.

If you recognize any of the preceding traits in yourself, work for self-change or stay out of the retail business.

WHOLESALE

If you don't like dealing with people you might be better off by selling wholesale. You still have to deal with people, but you'll be dealing with other businesspeople like yourself.

There are some drawbacks to wholesale trade. First, expect a smaller profit margin unless you have high volume sales. Second, the demand schedules (fulfilling your orders on time) will be vital to your business viability. You have to be able to produce and/or deliver the goods on time!

If you have a small operation, such as working from your kitchen on weekends, you might not have the volume to offer for wholesale trade. Most of the profit in wholesale trade comes from sales volume rather than item pricing. If this isn't your full-time occupation, wholesale might not be for you.

OTHER ALTERNATIVES

Many other avenues of business are available. Selling goods by consignment works for some people. It offers the advantage that somebody else actually sells the products. The disadvantage is all the paperwork required to keep track of where all your goods are being sold, how many, etc.

The most popular route for most people is at the community level. Flea markets, garage sales, and farmer's markets are profitable avenues for the right people. Some people even travel the circuit, attending and setting up shop in the various flea markets in an area. Two disadvantages with these operations are time and cost. These can be time-consuming and sometimes expensive. Also many of the people shopping at these events are looking for bargains. Your prices must be low to attract customers, sometimes unrealistically so. If you aren't making a profit, you aren't in business.

Even if you are operating at a profit, it is still a good idea to take inventory and assess your situation and marketing techniques on a monthly basis.

STARTING A BUSINESS

You'll probably have a number of questions about successfully starting a business. Fortunately, professional help is available.

Many chambers of commerce offer advice to area entrepreneurs. They might or might not be of much assistance depending on the circumstances, but they will be of no assistance if you don't ask them for help.

Another resource is your county extension agent. Extension services are linked to university business departments, and most offer helpful workshops for people interested in starting or running a business. Many of these have access to computer programs and can provide you with a marketing analysis, which could further improve your chances of success. People often have good ideas, but without market research they might be attempting the wrong strategies for their area. The fees for these services can be money well spent if they increase the chances of your success.

Don't overlook your local bookstore or library as an excellent reference source. A world of professional advice is at your fingertips through books.

Finally, don't be afraid to talk to others in the business. Avoid talking to direct competitors; they might try to discourage you or sabotage your efforts. Talk to people in the business. See how they are making out. This will give you a more realistic idea of what to expect and what to avoid when you open your doors for business.

Set realistic goals for yourself. It is highly unlikely that you will become a millionaire overnight, nor is being your own boss a ticket to easy street. Most people who work for themselves actually have to work harder than those who work for hourly wages. Remember, the success or failure of your business depends on you and you alone. The time and attention that you devote to your business can be vital to its success or failure, especially in its embryonic stage.

You can have a successful business, but you are going to have to work for it. If you are a person who believes in luck, you'd be better off playing the lottery. Business requires work, not luck.

BUSINESS ETHICS

Some people get so caught up in the competitive aspect of business and in making a buck that they forget the necessity of having a moral code of conduct. Ethics are especially important in business.

One of the best rules for success in business is the same rule for success in your personal life. It is the Golden Rule, "Do unto others as you would have them do unto you." If you practice the Golden Rule in your daily business, people will notice, word of mouth will attract more customers, and you are certain to get repeat sales.

If, however, you rip people off, they will also notice, and word of mouth can destroy your business. It really cannot be overemphasized: If you treat your customers in the same manner that you would like to be treated, you are going to keep those customers and attract new ones. Make your customers feel important—after all, they really are important to you.

Attitude

Your attitude reveals more than your personality. It is often a direct correlation to your business success (or lack of it). If you really are in business only to make money, then perhaps you should take a job at the U.S. Mint instead. Not just the things you say, but the way you act will affect your dealings with the general public.

Greed is unbecoming. Nobody even wants to buy from someone with that kind of attitude. Greedy people are rarely successful in business, and even when they are, they rarely find any real satisfaction in their success. Greed is not only bad morals, it's bad business.

Pricing Fluctuations

Sometimes prices have to be changed, but rapid fluctuations in your prices (especially upward) can be a source of concern or alarm to your customers. Customers will understand if you explain to them a need for price increases. But if they think that you are just padding prices to fatten your own wallet, customers won't be so forgiving.

FAMILY AFFAIR

A family business can be a wonderful thing, but there are pitfalls. Don't expect small children to handle great responsibilities. Be careful not to overwork family members, and never take anyone for granted. Pay the going rate, and be generous with bonuses for a job well done.

Some people think that because someone is a family member, that individual should work for free or for reduced wages. Such an attitude is bad for morale, hurtful to intra-familial relationships, and can ultimately affect your business adversely.

Also, don't discriminate against your family. Some firms bend over backwards to try to prove to their other employees that they don't show favoritism; sometimes they even discriminate against their own family. That is sheer nonsense! Nepotism doesn't deserve the bad rap that it has. It is all right to play favorites, provided you do not alienate other workers in the process or reward family members unfairly.

Keep family arguments out of the workplace. Your problems are best left at home. And don't permit business problems to interfere with family relationships. Your family is more important than any business! Finally, make it the policy that business be conducted as a business and home be conducted as a home.

Appendix

Sources of Supplies

MANY OF THE ITEMS you need to make your own potpourris, colognes, soaps, and other scented products will be available locally. Often it can mean a real savings to buy from a local store rather than through a mail-order specialty house. However, if you can't find what you need locally, you might find it helpful to shop by mail.

MAIL-ORDER SUPPLIERS

The following is a partial listing of mail-order supply companies that offer products useful for creating any of the projects contained in this book.

BUTTERICK PATTERN SERVICE
Box 1552, Altoona, PA 16603
Patterns for sewing projects, sachet pillows, rag dolls.

CRAFT KING, INC.
P.O. Box 90637, Lakeland, FL 33804
Craft supplies, sewing patterns.

HERRSCHNER'S
Steven's Point, WI 54481
Cloth, candle yarn, sewing patterns

INDIANA BOTANIC GARDENS
P.O. Box 5, Hammond, IN 46325
America's largest supplier of herbs and essential oils.

POURETTE
P.O. Box 15220, Seattle, WA 98115
Soap making supplies, candle making supplies, other craft items.

EARTH HERBS
40 N. 1st Street, Ventura, CA 93001
Herbs, extracts, essential oils.

FLOWER ESSENCE SERVICES
P.O. Box 1769, Nevada City, CA 95959
Herbal oils, floral oils.

KAUNAI FLOWER PERFUMES
P.O. Box 929H, Kalaheo, HI 96741
Tropical scents.

LITTLE SHEPHERD'S
9658E W. Chatfield Avenue, Littleton, CO 80123
Dried flowers, herbs, candle making and soap making supplies.

NATIVE SCENTS HERBAL INCENSE
Box 573, Taos, NM 87571
Incense, herbs, and botanicals.

OLD AMISH HERBAL
4141 Iris St. N., St. Petersburg, FL 33703
Essential oils, soap making supplies

RAVEN'S NEST
4539 Iroquois Trail, Duluth, GA 30136
Essential oils, spices, herbs.

SUNFEATHER HERBAL SOAP CO.
Rt. 3, Potsdam, NY 13676
Herbal powders, soap supplies.

VARNEY'S CHEMIST LADEN
c/o Fredericksburg Herb Farm
310 E. Main, Fredericksburg, TX 78624
Dried flowers, herbs, essential oils

TOM THUMB WORKSHOPS
Mappsville, VA 23407-0357
Potpourri supplies, spices, containers.

GOODWIN GREEK GARDENS
Box 83, Williams, OR 97544
Dried flowers, herbs.

ORIGINAL SWISS AROMATICS
P.O. Box 606, San Rafael, CA 94915
Essential oils, floral oils.

PENN HERB
603 N. 2nd Street, Philadelphia, PA 19123
Herbs, essential oils.

THE PEPPERMILL
8625 S. Market Place, Oak Creek, WI 53154
Potpourri supplies, essential oils, spices.

CAPRILANDS
Coventry, CT 06238
Potpourri supplies, herbs.

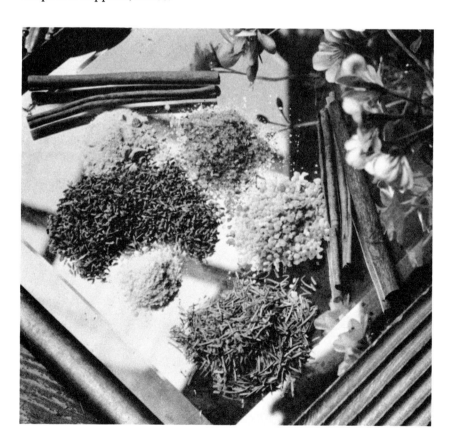

MAIL-ORDER PLANTS

If you want to grow your own flowers and herbs for potpourris, you can contact a number of companies that supply plants. Most nurseries will ship plants in the spring or fall only, so plan accordingly. Many of the plants grown for potpourri can be grown indoors on sunny windowsills; others are best grown in the garden.

Some companies charge a small fee for their catalogs. Write first for information.

BLUESTONE PERENNIALS
7247 Middleridge Road, Madison, OH 44057
An excellent source of quality perennial flowers and herbs.

BOUNTIFUL RIDGE NURSERIES
P.O. Box 250, Princess Anne, MD 21853
Fruits and flowers.

BROOKSIDE WILDFLOWERS
Rt. 3, Box 740, Boone, NC 28607
Wildflowers.

HENRY FIELD'S
Shenandoah, IA 51602
Roses, flowers, fruits.

LOGEE'S GREENHOUSE
North Street, Danielson, CT 06239
An excellent source of exotic and tropical houseplants. Logee's is *open all year round* so you can order houseplants as needed, not just in the spring or fall.

NATIVE GARDENS
Rt. 1, Box 494, Greenback, TN 37742
Specialize in wildflowers

ROCK SPRAY NURSERY
P.O. Box 693, Truro, MA 02666
Heather and rock garden flowers.

ROSES OF TODAY & YESTERDAY
802 Brown's Valley Road, Watsonville, CA 95076
Roses, old-time varieties and new.

STARK BROS. NURSERY
Louisiana, MO 63353
Fruits, lilacs, roses.

Index